TOP TRAILS™

Great Smoky Mountains National Park

MUST-DO HIKES FOR EVERYONE

TOP TRAILS™

Great Smoky Mountains National Park

MUST-DO HIKES FOR EVERYONE

Written by

Johnny Molloy

 WILDERNESS PRESS ... *on the trail since 1967*

Top Trails Great Smoky Mountains National Park: Must-Do Hikes for Everyone

1st EDITION 2012

ISBN 978-0-89997-677-8
Manufactured in the United States of America

Published by: **Wilderness Press**
               Keen Communications
               PO Box 43673
               Birmingham, AL 35243
               (800) 443-7227
               info@wildernesspress.com
               www.wildernesspress.com

Visit our website for a complete listing of our books and for ordering information.
Distributed by Publishers Group West

Cover photo: (*main*) Gregory Bald (Trail 4); (*inset*) trillium

SAFETY NOTICE: Although Wilderness Press and the author have made every attempt to ensure that the information in this book is accurate at press time, they are not responsible for any loss, damage, injury, or inconvenience that may occur to anyone while using this book. You are responsible for your own safety and health while in the wilderness. The fact that a trail is described in this book does not mean that it will be safe for you. Be aware that trail conditions can change from day to day. Always check local conditions, know your own limitations, and consult a map.

The Top Trails™ Series

Wilderness Press

When Wilderness Press published *Sierra North* in 1967, no other trail guide like it existed for the Sierra backcountry. The first run of 2,800 copies sold out in less than two months and its success heralded the beginning of Wilderness Press. Since we were founded more than 40 years ago, we have expanded our territories to cover California, Alaska, Hawaii, the U.S. Southwest, the Pacific Northwest, New England, and Canada. And most recently, we have pushed our boundaries into the Southeast.

Wilderness Press continues to publish comprehensive, accurate, and readable outdoor books. Hikers, backpackers, kayakers, skiers, snowshoers, climbers, cyclists, and trail runners rely on Wilderness Press for accurate outdoor adventure information.

Top Trails

In its Top Trails guides, Wilderness Press has paid special attention to organization so that you can find the perfect hike each and every time. Whether you're looking for a steep trail to test yourself on or a walk in the park, a romantic waterfall or a city view, Top Trails will lead you there.

Each Top Trails guide contains trails for everyone. The trails selected provide a sampling of the best that the region has to offer. These are the "must-do" hikes, walks, runs, and bike rides, with every feature of the area represented.

Every book in the Top Trails series offers:

- The Wilderness Press commitment to accuracy and reliability
- Ratings and rankings for each trail
- Distances and approximate times
- Easy-to-follow trail notes
- Map and permit information

Great Smoky Mountains National Park

Sevierville

411

Ch 2: Tremont and Elkmont Area

Pigeon Forge

441

Ch 1: Abrams Creek and Cades Cove Area

Maryville

321

321 Townsend

Cades Cove

Tremont

Ch 5:

Chilowee

Ch 4: Twentymile and Fontana Lake Area

GREAT SMOKY
MOUNTAINS
NATIONAL
PARK

129

Calderwood

TENNESSEE
NORTH CAROLINA

Tapoco

28

Fontana Lake

Fontana Village

28

74 19

129

CHEROKEE
NATIONAL
FOREST

Cosby

40 Hartford

Ch 3: Mount Le Conte, Greenbrier, and Cosby Area

32

Ch 6: Smokemont, Cataloochee, and Big Creek Area

Gatlinburg

301

40

TENNESSEE
NORTH CAROLINA

PISGAH
NATIONAL
FOREST

Deep, Forney, and Noland Creeks Area

441

Maggie
Valley

19

Cherokee

19

Bryson
City

74

74

N

441

0   2   4   6 miles

0   2   4   6 kilometers

23

Great Smoky Mountains National Park Trails

TRAIL NUMBER AND NAME	Page	Difficulty -12345+	Length in Miles	Type	Backpacking	Dayhiking	Horses	Child Friendly
1. Abrams Creek and Cades Cove Area								
1 Pine Mountain Loop	27	2–3	8.1	Loop	Backpacking	Dayhiking	Horses	
2 Abrams Falls via Abrams Creek Ranger Station	33	3	11.0	Out & Back	Backpacking	Dayhiking		
3 Abrams Falls via Cades Cove	39	2	5.0	Out & Back		Dayhiking		
4 Gregory Bald via Gregory Ridge	43	4	11.0	Out & Back	Backpacking	Dayhiking		
5 Oliver Cabin via Rich Mountain Loop Trail	49	1–2	2.8	Out & Back		Dayhiking	Horses	Child Friendly
6 Spence Field and Russell Field Loop	55	4–5	13.0	Loop	Backpacking	Dayhiking	Horses	
7 Rocky Top via Lead Cove	61	5	11.6	Out & Back	Backpacking	Dayhiking	Horses	
8 Finley Cane Loop	65	3	8.8	Loop		Dayhiking	Horses	
2. Tremont and Elkmont Area								
9 Lynn Camp Prong Cascades	81	1	0.8	Out & Back		Dayhiking		Child Friendly
10 Buckhorn Gap via Meigs Creek	87	2–3	6.8	Out & Back		Dayhiking		
11 Walker Sisters Place via Little Greenbrier	91	2	5.0	Out & Back		Dayhiking		
12 Cucumber Gap Loop	97	2–3	5.6	Loop		Dayhiking		
13 Little River Hike	103	3	7.8	Out & Back	Backpacking	Dayhiking		
14 The Chimney Tops	107	3	4.0	Out & Back		Dayhiking		
15 Silers Bald via Clingmans Dome	111	3	9.6	Out & Back	Backpacking	Dayhiking		
3. Mount Le Conte, Greenbrier, and Cosby Area								
16 Charlies Bunion	127	3–4	8.0	Out & Back	Backpacking	Dayhiking		
17 Alum Cave Bluff	131	2–3	4.6	Out & Back		Dayhiking		
18 Rainbow Falls	137	2–3	5.4	Out & Back		Dayhiking		
19 Brushy Mountain via Grotto Falls	141	4	6.6	Out & Back		Dayhiking		
20 Injun Creek from Greenbrier	147	2–3	6.4	Out & Back	Backpacking	Dayhiking		
21 Ramsey Cascades	153	4	8.0	Out & Back		Dayhiking		
22 Albright Grove	157	3	6.7	Loop		Dayhiking		
23 Maddron Bald Loop	163	4–5	17.3	Loop	Backpacking			
24 Sutton Ridge Overlook	171	2	3.6	Out & Back		Dayhiking		Child Friendly
25 Mount Cammerer via Low Gap	175	5	11.2	Out & Back		Dayhiking		

TYPE	USES & ACCESS	TERRAIN
Loop	Dayhiking — Horses	Mountain — Stream
Out & Back	Backpacking — Child Friendly	Summit — Waterfall
Point-to-Point		Ridgeline — Lake

DIFFICULTY
-12345+
less   more

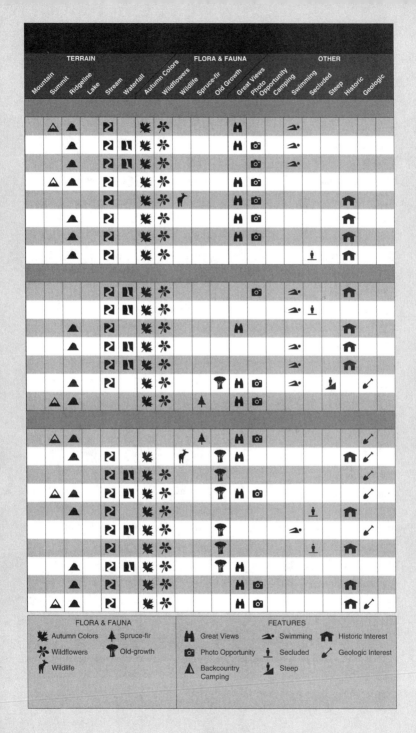

TERRAIN · FLORA & FAUNA · OTHER

Mountain · Summit · Ridgeline · Lake · Stream · Waterfall · Autumn Colors · Wildflowers · Wildlife · Spruce-fir · Old Growth · Great Views · Photo Opportunity · Camping · Swimming · Secluded · Steep · Historic · Geologic

FLORA & FAUNA

- Autumn Colors
- Wildflowers
- Wildlife
- Spruce-fir
- Old-growth

FEATURES

- Great Views
- Photo Opportunity
- Backcountry Camping
- Swimming
- Secluded
- Steep
- Historic Interest
- Geologic Interest

Great Smoky Mountains National Park Trails

TRAIL NUMBER AND NAME	Page	Difficulty -12345+	Length in Miles	Type	Backpacking	Dayhiking	Horses	Child Friendly
4. Twentymile and Fontana Lake Area								
26 Twentymile Loop	191	2	7.6	Loop	Backpacking	Dayhiking	Horses	
27 Gregory Bald Loop	197	4	15.5	Loop	Backpacking		Horses	
28 Shuckstack from Twentymile Ranger Station	205	3	11.0	Out & Back	Backpacking	Dayhiking		
29 Lost Cove Loop	211	3–4	11.5	Loop	Backpacking	Dayhiking		
30 Fontana Lake Hike	217	3	13.3	Point-to-Point	Backpacking	Dayhiking	Horses	
31 Ruins of Proctor	225	1	2.0	Out & Back	Backpacking	Dayhiking		Child Friendly
5. Deep, Forney, and Noland Creeks Area								
32 Goldmine Loop	241	2	3.2	Loop	Backpacking	Dayhiking	Horses	
33 Whiteoak Branch Loop	247	2	8.8	Loop	Backpacking	Dayhiking	Horses	
34 Indian Creek and Sunkota Ridge Loop	253	3	12.0	Loop	Backpacking	Dayhiking	Horses	
35 Falls Loop of Deep Creek	259	1–2	2.4	Loop		Dayhiking		Child Friendly
36 Newton Bald Loop	265	5	22.5	Loop	Backpacking		Horses	
37 Fork Ridge Loop	273	5	20.1	Loop	Backpacking		Horses	
38 Forney Creek Loop	281	5	19.4	Loop	Backpacking		Horses	
39 Andrews Bald	287	2	3.6	Out & Back		Dayhiking		Child Friendly
6. Smokemont, Cataloochee, and Big Creek Area								
40 Smokemont Loop	303	2	6.0	Loop		Dayhiking		
41 Cabin Flats Loop	309	4	17.4	Loop	Backpacking		Horses	
42 Hyatt Ridge Loop	315	3	7.6	Loop		Dayhiking	Horses	
43 Flat Creek Falls	321	2	3.8	Out & Back		Dayhiking		Child Friendly
44 Hemphill Bald Hike	327	3–4	9.6	Out & Back	Backpacking			
45 Big Fork Ridge Loop	333	3	9.1	Loop	Backpacking	Dayhiking	Horses	
46 Pretty Hollow Gap Loop	339	4–5	19.1	Loop	Backpacking		Horses	
47 Boogerman Loop	345	3	7.5	Loop		Dayhiking		
48 Little Cataloochee Church	351	2	4.0	Out & Back		Dayhiking		
49 Mount Sterling via Mount Sterling Gap	357	3	5.4	Out & Back	Backpacking	Dayhiking	Horses	
50 Midnight Hole and Mouse Creek Falls	363	2	4.0	Out & Back		Dayhiking	Horses	

TYPE
- ⟳ Loop
- ↗ Out & Back
- ↘ Point-to-Point

DIFFICULTY
- 1 2 3 4 5 +
less   more

USES & ACCESS
- Dayhiking
- Backpacking
- Horses
- Child Friendly

TERRAIN
- Mountain
- Summit
- Ridgeline
- Stream
- Waterfall
- Lake

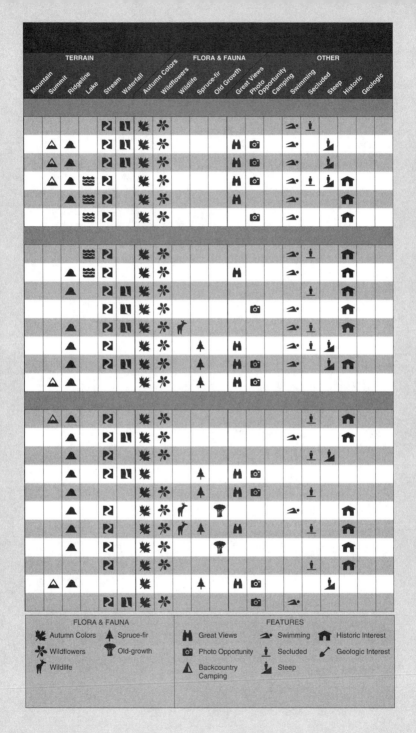

Contents

CHAPTER 1
Abrams Creek and Cades Cove Area . . . 15

Using Top Trails™

Organization of Top Trails

Top Trails is designed to make identifying the perfect trail easy and enjoyable, and to make every outing a success and a pleasure. With this book you'll find it's a snap to find the right trail, whether you're planning a major hike or just a sociable stroll with friends.

The Region

Each Top Trails begins with a regional map (pages vi–vii), displaying the entire area covered by the guide and providing an overview of the geography. The map is clearly marked to show which chapter covers which area.

After the regional map comes the master trails table (pages viii–xi), which lists every trail covered in the guide. Here you'll find a concise description, basic information, and highlighted features, all indispensable when planning an outing. A quick reading of the regional map and trails table will give you a good overview of the entire region covered by the book.

Navigating the Region

GSMNP
Regional Map
pages vi–vii

GSMNP Trails Table
pages viii–xi

The Areas

The region covered in each book is divided into areas, with each chapter corresponding to one area in the region. Each area chapter starts with information to help you choose and enjoy a trail every time out. Use the table of contents or the regional map to identify an area of interest, then turn to the area chapter to find the following:

- An overview of the area's parks and trails, including park and permit information
- An area map showing all trail locations
- A trail features table providing trail-by-trail details
- Trail summaries highlighting each trail's specific features

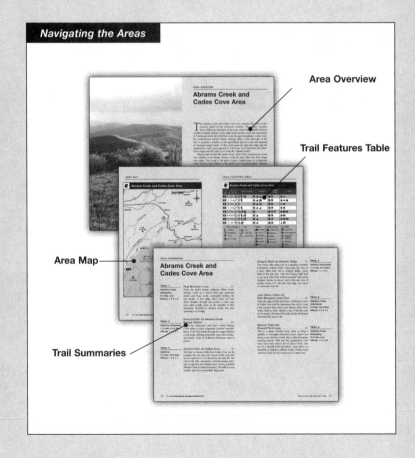

The Trails

The basic building block of the Top Trails guide is the trail entry. Each one is arranged to make finding and following the trail as simple as possible, with all pertinent information presented in this easy-to-follow format:

- A detailed trail map
- Trail descriptors covering difficulty, length, and other essential data
- A written trail description
- Trail milestones providing easy-to follow, turn-by-turn trail directions

Some trail descriptions offer additional information:

- An elevation profile
- Trail options
- Trail highlights

In the margins of the trail entries, keep your eyes open for graphic icons that signal features mentioned in the text.

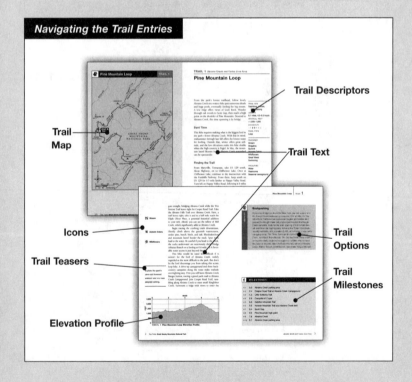

Choosing a Trail

Top Trails provides several different ways of choosing a trail, all presented in easy-to-read tables, charts, and maps.

Location

If you know in general where you want to go, Top Trails makes it easy to find the right trail in the right place. Each chapter begins with a large-scale map showing the starting point of every trail in that area.

Features

This guide describes the Top Trails of Great Smoky Mountains National Park, and each trail is chosen because it offers one or more features that make it appealing. Using the trail descriptors, summaries, and tables, you can quickly examine all the trails for the features they offer or seek a particular feature among the list of trails.

Best Time

Time of year and current conditions can be important factors in selecting the best trail. For example, an exposed low-elevation trail may be a riot of color in early spring, but an oven-baked taste of hell in midsummer. Wherever relevant, Top Trails identifies the best and worst conditions for the trails you plan to hike.

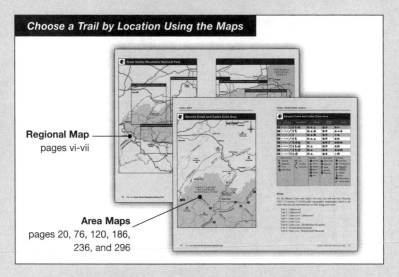

Choose a Trail by Location Using the Maps

Regional Map — pages vi-vii

Area Maps — pages 20, 76, 120, 186, 236, and 296

Difficulty

Every trail has an overall difficulty rating on a scale of 1 to 5, which takes into consideration length, elevation change, exposure, trail quality, etc., to create one (admittedly subjective) rating.

The ratings assume you are an able-bodied adult in reasonably good shape, using the trail for hiking. The ratings also assume normal weather conditions—clear and dry.

Readers should make an honest assessment of their own abilities and adjust time estimates accordingly. Also, rain, snow, heat, wind, and poor visibility can all affect your pace on even the easiest of trails.

Vertical Feet

Every trail description contains the approximate trail length and the overall elevation gain and loss over the course of the trail. It's important to use this figure when considering a hike; on average plan one hour for every 2 miles, and add an hour for every 1,000 feet you climb.

This important measurement is often underestimated by hikers when gauging the difficulty of a trail. The Top Trails measurement accounts for all elevation change, not simply the difference between the highest and lowest points, so that rolling terrain with lots of up and down will be identifiable.

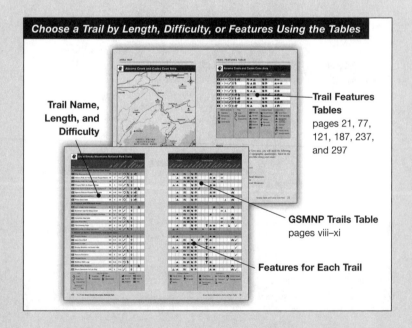

Choose a Trail by Length, Difficulty, or Features Using the Tables

Trail Name, Length, and Difficulty

Trail Features Tables
pages 21, 77, 121, 187, 237, and 297

GSMNP Trails Table
pages viii–xi

Features for Each Trail

Map Legend

Featured trail	▬ ▬ ▬ ▬ ▬ ▬ ▬ ▬	Point of interest	●
Alternate trail	– – – – – – – –	Bridge	⩲
Cross-country trail	··············	Tunnel	⌂
		Parking	🅿
Interstate	▬▬▬▬▬▬	Gate	●—●
Major road	▬▬▬▬▬▬	Ranger station	⌂
Minor road	————	Campground/campsite	▲
		Picnic area	⊼
Water body		Appalachian Trail	◈
River/creek	————	Mountain	▲
		Vista point	Ħ
State boundary	–·–·–·–·–	Waterfall	//
		Rapids/cascades	〿
Park/forest	▬▬▬▬	Building (can be any shape)	▮
		Interstate shields	40
		US Highway shields	441
North indicator	N ✦	State Highway shields	28

Top Trails Difficulty Ratings

1 A short trail, generally level, that can be completed in one hour or less.

2 A route of 1 to 3 miles, with some up and down, that can be completed in one to two hours.

3 A longer route, up to 5 miles, with uphill and/or downhill sections.

4 A long or steep route, perhaps more than 5 miles, or with climbs of more than 1,000 vertical feet.

5 The most severe route, both long and steep, more than 5 miles long with climbs of more than 1,000 vertical feet.

The calculation of vertical feet in the Top Trails books is accomplished by a combination of trail measurement and computer-aided estimation. For routes that begin and end at the same spot—i.e., loop or out-and-back—the vertical gain exactly matches the vertical descent; simply halve the figure listed for the trail With a point-to-point route, the vertical gain and loss will most likely differ, but the figure listed is the overall figure.

Finally, all Trail Entries include an elevation profile, an easy means for visualizing the topography of the route. These profiles graphically depict the elevation throughout the length of the trail.

Introduction to Great Smoky Mountains National Park

I have been hiking the Smokies since the early 1980s and have had a Smokies guide in print since 1995, with multiple updated and improved editions. Preparing this guide for Wilderness Press gave me the chance to entirely rehike all the trails and write a new guide to what I think is the most beautiful place on the planet. You will find this easy-access reference-type book a marked improvement.

Though I have spent more than 750 nights backpacking in the Smokies and countless other times dayhiking, any chance to return to the park lets me rediscover and appreciate the crown jewel of the Southern Appalachians. Writing this book meant more reasons to get back to the park where I cut my outdoor teeth.

And what a park it is: more than 900 miles of trails, 500,000 acres of land, and some of the largest stands of old-growth forest in the East. The numbers of flora and fauna are just as impressive: 60 species of mammals, 50 species of fish, 200 species of birds, 1,600 species of flowering plants, 2,000 species of fungi, and more.

With the all taxa survey, an attempted cataloging of every living thing in the park, the sheer numbers and types of life cataloged keep rising. The park boasts numerous trees of record dimensions among the upward of 130 species that grow here. The diversity of ecosystems found in the Smokies is unmatched in any other temperate climate. Perhaps this is the reason for its impressive designation as both a national park and an international biosphere reserve.

Choosing the Smokies as a place to spend your free time is a wise decision. And yet the Smokies can be intimidating, especially for the first-time visitor. Not only is there a lot of land to see, but with more than 9 million guests annually, the Great Smoky Mountains National Park is the most visited national park in the American system—quite intimidating indeed. Thus, this book was conceived to make the majesty of the Smokies more accessible to visitors.

With so much land and so many people, discovering the beauty and solitude of this national park can be a hit-or-miss proposition. Where are the spectacular vistas? Where are the waterfalls and the old settlers' cabins? Where can I find solitude? Leaving it all to chance doesn't offer good odds for your all-too-brief vacation from the rat race. Weeks spent daydreaming of your fleeting slice of freedom could culminate in a three-hour driving marathon or a noisy walk up a crowded trail. Fortunately, with this book, and a little bit of planning and forethought, you can make the most of your time in the Smokies.

This book presents a variety of hikes for you to choose from. The majority of the hikes steer you toward infrequently visited areas, giving you the opportunity to enjoy your time on the trail instead of behind someone's car. These hikes offer solitude to maximize your Smoky Mountains experience. However, as the subtitle of this book suggests, there are some "must-do" hikes that are popular. Consequently, portions of hikes traverse popular and potentially crowded areas. Each hike has a described "best time" that will help you manage the trails to your advantage.

The dayhikes offered here fall into one of two categories: out-and-back or loop. Out-and-back hikes take you to a particular rewarding destination and back on the same trail. The return trip allows you to see everything from the opposite vantage point. You may notice more minute features the second go-round, and retracing your steps at a different time of day can give the same trail a surprisingly different character.

To some, however, a return trip on the same trail isn't as enjoyable. Some hikers just can't stand the thought of covering the same ground twice, not with hundreds of untrodden Smokies miles awaiting them. Loop hikes avoid this. The loop hikes in this book are generally longer than the out-and-back hikes, but a bigger challenge can reap bigger rewards.

Dayhiking is the best and most popular way to "break into" the Smokies backcountry, but for those with the inclination, this book also offers some overnight hikes. There are 102 designated backcountry sites and shelters available for those who want to capture the changing moods of the mountains. The length of these hikes, three days and two nights, are perfect for the weekend backpacker. Longer trips are also available for those with more time.

A permit is required for overnight stays in the backcountry. Certain campsites may be reserved in advance. Permits are available at visitor centers or by calling (865) 436-1231. Food storage cables have been installed at backcountry campsites. Please use them—you get to keep your food and it keeps wild bears wild. Bears that get too used to human food often have to be exterminated.

When visiting the Smokies, it's a great temptation to remain in your car, in part because auto tours—including one end of the famed Blue Ridge

Parkway—abound. While auto touring is a great way to get an overview of the park, it creates a barrier between you and the mountains. Windshield tourists, hoping for a glimpse of bears and other wildlife, often end up seeing the tail end of the car in front of them. And while roadside overlooks offer easy views, the drone of traffic and lack of effort in reaching the views can make them less than inspirational. The Smokies were made for hiking.

The wilderness experience can unleash your mind and body, allowing you to relax and find peace and quiet. It also enables you to catch glimpses of beauty and splendor: a deer crashing through the underbrush as it clambers up a mountainside, the cabin remnants of early settlers who scrabbled out a living among these woods, or a spectacular waterfall crashing above and below a trail. Out in these woods, you can let your mind roam free, go where it pleases. A climate-controlled automobile does *not* allow such wandering.

The Smokies are a wild and beautiful place. I hope you will get out and enjoy what they have to offer.

Geography and Topography

The topography of the Great Smoky Mountains results from the weathering of one of the oldest mountain ranges in the world—the Appalachians. The Smokies, however, are the highest, wildest range in the entire chain, with more than 30 continuous miles above 5,000 feet, an outlying mountain massif unmatched anywhere east of the Mississippi. Elevations vary from 6,642 feet at Clingmans Dome (a scant 40 feet lower than Mount Mitchell, the highest point in the East) down to the mouth of Abrams Creek, under 900 feet. This vertical variation is one of the reasons for the incredible diversity of life found within its boundaries.

From the Smokies emerges many a tributary for the Tennessee River. The Little River drains the high country directly into the Tennessee, while others, such the Oconaluftee River, feed bigger tributaries, namely the Pigeon and Little Tennessee Rivers, which in turn flow into the Tennessee River. The Little Tennessee River is dammed in a series of finger lakes (Fontana, Cheoah, and Calderwood) that form the Smokies' southern boundary.

The dominant landform is a high, continuous ridge extending east-west from one end of the Smokies to the other. In addition to dividing river drainages, it also forms the boundary line between North Carolina and Tennessee. Shoulder ridges, like ribs protruding from a backbone, extend from the state line ridge and separate steep yet deeply wooded valleys cut by eons of precipitation. The Smokies boasts more than 2,100 miles of streams within its 800-square-mile confines.

Flora

The flora of the Smokies from low to high replicates a biological journey up the Appalachian Mountains from Georgia to Maine. Upward of 130 tree species are native to the park. It is not just the beautiful trees and wildflowers that get attention, the Smokies also have amazing arrays of more humble yet biologically important plants from mosses to fungi.

The diverse plant mosaic blends and separates depending on elevation, precipitation, and exposure. In the park's lower reaches grow Southern temperate woodlands, an agglomeration of hardwoods from hickory, sourwood, and sassafras in drier areas to elm, maple, and ash in moister soils. Along the streams, towering white pines, black birch, and imperiled hemlock reign over thickets of rhododendron.

The great cove hardwood forests, where sheltered valleys harbor deep soils, are where tree giants can be found. Dominated by tulip trees, along with buckeye and basswood, the cove hardwoods rise to immense heights, creating a 150- to 200-foot canopy in cool moist hollows.

Drier, well-drained or south-facing ridges have xeric woods of Virginia pine, chestnut oak, and mountain laurel, along with a host of lesser oaks. Climbing higher, the vegetation morphs into northern hardwoods, such as yellow birch, beech, and cherry. Rise still higher and you get into the spruce-fir woodlands, where evergreens form a mosaic of plant life found in New England or Canada. The forest cloaks the highest mantles of the park, and of that only around 13,000 acres of pure spruce-fir, a relic of a colder time. The last of the ice ages pushed this northern evergreen ecosystem south, and when the earth warmed again, the forest clung atop old Smoky in a climate still favorable for it. This has, in effect, created sky islands of plants and animals whose normal range is far removed from Dixie.

Together these forest types, blending and intermingling, comprise arguably the most diverse biological life in earth's temperate climes. But the trees are the most visible of the plants, for each of these forests has accompanying lesser known and seen plant forms that carpet the Smokies. The number of plant species is always rising as the well-researched park continually reveals new life-forms. The all taxa survey, an attempt to catalog every life-form in the park, has resulted in an explosion of heretofore undocumented species.

Fauna

The rich vegetation environment and large amount of wild land support an impressive array of mammals—more than 60 species. The black bear thrives in the Smokies, with an estimated 1,500 species roaming within its boundaries, nearly two per square mile, arguably the densest concentration of bruins in North America. However, the population follows the yearly rise and fall of mast—berries, acorns, and the like. When the lower regions of the park were populated, unregulated hunting nearly drove the black bear from the Smokies, but the beasts hung on, and their numbers inside the park grew and stabilized. This park population of *Ursus americanus* creates a core from which surrounding lands also harbor plenty of bruins. Species management by wildlife agencies and people simply learning better how to live with bears has helped too. And since wild animals know no boundaries or borders, the greater populations outside the park keep the numbers of bears up throughout the Southern Appalachians. The state of Tennessee is thought to have more bears now than any time during the last century.

Extensive efforts have been made to keep black bears wild in the park. Gone are the days of roadside feedings. Education and bearproof garbage cans in the frontcountry and bearproof food-hanging cables in the back-country have reduced negative "people-bear" interactions.

Elk have been successfully reintroduced into the park, beginning in 2001, and their bugling can be heard in Cataloochee. The beasts will often be seen as well, grazing the meadows. The populations are reproducing, and the reintroduction is a resounding success. A red wolf reintroduction failed, but otters were successfully brought back and can now be found in many a Smokies stream. Peregrine falcons again soar above the slopes of Mount Le Conte after a park effort to restore this noble bird.

White-tailed deer are the animal you are most likely to see in the park. They can be found in woods and especially historically cleared areas such as Cades Cove. A quiet hiker may also witness turkeys on wooded hillsides or in clearings. Furtive bobcats can sometimes be spotted crossing trails. Raccoons are occasionally spotted in the wild and can be a nuisance at backcountry campsites. Coyotes are found throughout the park, but will usually spot you before you spot them.. A bounding tan tail disappearing into the distance will likely comprise a sighting of this critter, which effectively replaced the extirpated red wolf. Don't be surprised if you observe beavers or muskrats in Smokies streams. Beaver can be found in the lowermost, slowest park waters.

The Smokies critters reflect the varied forest types. In the high country, red squirrels will chatter at you from evergreen boughs. Overhead, birds, including pileated woodpeckers and red-tailed hawks, will ply the forest for food. The Eastern screech owl will emit its goose-bump-raising calls. While hiking you may be startled by a ruffed grouse blasting from its camouflaged trailside locale. Songbirds native to the north and south find a home in the park. Other migrants come and go with the seasons. Birding is a popular pastime in the park and can add to a hike.

The main game fish in the Smokies is cold water trout. The brook trout is the only native to the Smokies. Technically, the brook is not a true trout, but a char. Brooks prefer cold, clear waters and are primarily relegated to higher elevation streams, though the park service continues to restore brook habitat. Brook trout exclusively occupy 97 miles of trout streams in the park. Rainbow trout were introduced the park following logging, and have displaced native brook in many streams. Brown trout, a European native also introduced following logging, are found in quieter, stiller water, often in deep pools. Smallmouth bass and rock bass occupy the warmer, slower, and lower park streams. Beyond the game species, more than four dozen other fish species ply the Smokies waters. Some, such as the Smoky madtom, are quite rare, and make the case for protecting the Smokies.

Interestingly, the Smokies may have more life mass in salamanders than any other vertebrate. At least 24 kinds have been found here. Biologists come from all over the world to study them. It is just one more example of how the life in these mountains lives up to its national park status.

When to Go

The Smokies have a somewhat undeserved reputation of being over-crowded. Yes, the roadways of the Smokies are crowded during summer, on warm season weekends, and on holidays. The roads are also busy during the October leaf-viewing season. However, get a quarter mile from a trailhead on a hiking trail, and you will experience solitude. Busy trails—and there are some—are noted in the narratives.

Great Smoky Mountains National Park is a four-season destination. Hikers with well-thought-out plans can easily execute their treks beyond the obvious busy times. Try to hike midweek and just before or after major holidays. Spring is a great time. Fall can be great, too, but avoid October weekends. Solitude can be found anytime during winter. As far as busy trails, try to hike them early in the morning, or later in the evening. Iffy weather, such a 50-percent or more chance of rain, often keeps the crowds away. Avoid busy trails on nice weather weekends.

Weather and Seasons

The Smoky Mountains offer four distinct seasons for the hiker's enjoyment, but sometimes it seems all four are going on at once, depending on your location and elevation. Before your visit is over, you will probably see a little bit of everything.

The adjacent chart is from Gatlinburg, Tennessee, located just outside the park. Expect temperatures in the higher portions of the park to be 10 to 15 degrees cooler.

Average High and Low Temperature by Month, Gatlinburg, Tennessee					
	JAN	FEB	MAR	APR	MAY	JUNE
High	48°	52°	61°	69°	76°	82°
Low	25°	26°	33°	39°	49°	57°
	JULY	AUG	SEPT	OCT	NOV	DEC
High	85°	84°	79°	70°	60°	51°
Low	62°	60°	54°	42°	33°	28°

Be prepared for a wide range of temperatures and conditions, no matter the season. As a rule of thumb, the temperature decreases about three degrees with every 1,000 feet of elevation gained. The Smokies are also the wettest place in the South. The park's higher elevations can receive upward of 90 inches of precipitation a year.

Spring, the most variable season, takes six weeks to reach the park's highest elevations. You may encounter both winter- and summer-like weather during April and May, often in the same day. As the weather warms, thunderstorms become more frequent. Summer days typically start clear, but as the day heats up, clouds build, often culminating in a heavy shower. Fall, the driest season, comes to the peaks in early September, working its way downhill, the reverse pattern of spring; warm days and cool nights are interspersed with less-frequent wet periods.

Winter presents the Smokies at their most challenging. Frontal systems sweep through the region, with alternately cloudy and sunny days, though cloudy days are most frequent. No permanent snowpack exists in the high country, though areas higher than 5,000 feet receive five feet of snow or more per year. The high country can see bitterly cold temperature readings during this time. When venturing in the Smokies, it's a good idea to carry clothes for all weather extremes.

Trail Selection

Four criteria were used during the selection of trails for this guide. Only the premier dayhikes and overnight backpacking trips are included, based upon most beautiful scenery, unique Smoky Mountain features, ease of access, and diversity of experience. Some of the selected trails are very popular; others are used infrequently. If you are fortunate enough to complete all the hikes in this book, you will gain a comprehensive appreciation for the complex beauty of one of the world's most scenic and intact ecosystems in the temperate climate.

Key Features

Top Trails books contain information about features for each trail, such as old-growth trees, waterfalls, great views, and more. Great Smoky Mountains National Park is blessed with an incredible diversity of terrain and associated flora and fauna—no matter your interests, you're sure to find a trail to match them. Hikes range throughout the vast variety of ecosystems, from the spruce-fir high country to the old-growth forests to the verdant streams valleys where waterfalls tumble still deeper into the back of beyond. Those who love a view will find plenty of rock outcrops, balds, fire towers, and other vista points where rewarding views can be had. Photographers will be glad we live in the age of the digital camera, as they can shoot limitless shots of showy spring wildflowers and vibrant fall-color panoramas.

Campgrounds are situated throughout the park and make great base-camps for hikers. Backcountry campsites allow hikers to extend their trips beyond dayhiking. Anglers can toss a line in more than 2,000 miles of waters. Paddlers can ply the seasonal whitewater streams or enjoy the flat water of Fontana Lake. Swimming holes are abundant in the Smokies creeks. Wildlife can be seen in the meadows of Cades Cove and Cataloochee and other places between.

Multiple Uses

All the trails described in this guide are suitable for hiking. Many of the trails can also be enjoyed by equestrians, though the number of horseback enthusiasts in the Smokies is far outstripped by hikers. Very few trails, except for dedicated horse paths used by park concessionaires, have more than sporadic equestrian use. Just a short stretch of the Deep Creek Trail is open to bicycles. Two-wheel enthusiasts are otherwise relegated to sharing the roads, though Cades Cove Loop Road is closed to autos on certain days during the warm season. Paddlers and motorboaters are increasingly using watercraft to access the trails and campsites bordering Fontana Lake. Fishing is done along both park road streams and in the backcountry. A small number of cross-country ski enthusiasts use Clingmans Dome Road, closed during the winter, to enjoy the ample snow. As in most national parks, pets are not allowed on backcountry trails.

On the Trail

Every outing should begin with proper preparation, which usually takes only a few minutes. Even the easiest trail can turn up unexpected surprises. People seldom think about getting lost or injured, but unexpected things can and do happen. Simple precautions can make the difference between a good story and a dangerous situation.

Use the Top Trails ratings and descriptions to determine if a particular trail is a good match with your fitness and energy level, given current conditions and the time of year.

Have a Plan

Choose Wisely The first step to enjoying any trail is to match the trail to your abilities. It's no use overestimating your experience or fitness—know your abilities and limitations, and use the Top Trails difficulty rating that accompanies each trail.

Leave Word about Your Plans The most basic of precautions is leaving word of your intentions with friends or family. Many people will hike the backcountry their entire lives without ever relying on this safety net, but establishing this simple habit is free insurance.

It's best to leave specific information—location, trail name, intended time of travel—with a responsible person. If there is a registration process available, make use of it. If there is a ranger station, trail register, or park office, check in.

Prepare and Plan

- Know your abilities and your limitations.
- Leave word about your plans with family and friends.
- Know the area and the route.

Review the Route Before embarking on any hike, read the entire description and study the map. It isn't necessary to memorize every detail, but it is worthwhile to have a clear mental picture of the trail and the general area. If the trail or terrain are complex, augment the trail guide with a topographic map. Park maps, as well as current weather and trail condition information, are often available from local ranger and park stations.

Carry the Essentials

Proper preparation for any type of trail use includes gathering certain essential items to carry. Your trip checklist will vary according to trail choice and conditions.

Trail Essentials

- Dress to keep cool, but be ready for cold.
- Bring plenty of water and adequate food.

Clothing When the weather is good, light, comfortable clothing is the obvious choice. It's easy to believe that very little spare clothing is needed, but a prepared hiker has something tucked away for any emergency from a surprise shower to an unexpected overnight in a remote area.

Clothing includes proper footwear, essential for hiking and running trails. As a trail becomes more demanding, you will need footwear that performs. Running shoes are fine for many trails. If you will be carrying substantial weight or encountering sustained rugged terrain, step up to hiking boots.

The Smokies can be notoriously humid in summer. Hikers often sweat more than normal. Breathable, moisture-wicking clothes will help keep you cool and dry. In cooler weather, particularly when it's wet, carry water-proof outer garments and quick-drying undergarments (avoid cotton). The Smokies can be a rainy place. Unless the forecast calls for absolutely no chance of rain, bring a rain jacket or poncho. As general rule, whatever the conditions, bring layers that can be combined or removed to provide comfort and protection from the elements in a wide variety of conditions.

Water Never embark on a trail without carrying water. At all times, particularly in warm weather, adequate water is of key importance. Experts recommend at least two quarts of water per day, and when hiking in heat a gallon or more may be more appropriate. At the extreme, dehydration can be life threatening. More commonly, inadequate water brings fatigue and muscle aches.

For most outings, unless the day is very hot or the trail very long, you should plan to carry sufficient water for the entire trail. Unfortunately, in North America natural water sources are questionable, generally loaded with various risks: bacteria, viruses, and fertilizers.

Water Treatment If it's necessary to make use of trailside water, you should filter or treat it. There are three methods for treating water: boiling, chemical treatment, and filtering. Boiling is best, but often impractical—it requires a heat source, a pot, and time. Chemical treatments, available in sporting goods stores, handle some problems, including the troublesome *Giardia* parasite, but will not combat many artificial chemical pollutants. The preferred method is filtration, which removes *Giardia* and other contaminants and doesn't leave any unpleasant aftertaste.

If this hasn't convinced you to carry all the water you need, one final admonishment: be prepared for surprises. Water sources described in the text or on maps can change course or dry up completely. Never run your water bottle dry in expectation of the next source; fill up when water is available and always keep a little in reserve.

Food

While not as critical as water, food is energy and its importance shouldn't be underestimated. Avoid foods that are hard to digest, such as candy bars and potato chips. Carry high energy, fast-digesting foods: nutrition bars, dehydrated fruit, gorp, and jerky. Bring a little extra food—it's good protection against an outing that turns unexpectedly long, perhaps because of inclement weather or losing your way.

Useful but Less than Essential Items

Map and Compass (and the Know-How to Use Them) Many trails don't require much navigation, meaning a map and compass aren't always as essential as water or food—but it can be a close call. If the trail is remote or infrequently visited, a map and compass should be considered necessities.

A handheld GPS (Global Positioning System) receiver is also a useful trail companion, but is really no substitute for a map and compass. However, a GPS downloaded with topographic maps can be a real help. The hazard is batteries dying or the device otherwise becoming unusable. A map and compass don't require batteries.

Cell Phone Some ridges and areas near Gatlinburg have some level of cellular coverage. However, for most areas, especially in hollows and along streams, there is no phone service. In extreme circumstances, a cell phone can be a lifesaver. But don't depend on it; coverage is too unpredictable and batteries fail. And be sure that the occasion warrants the phone call—a blister doesn't justify a call to search-and-rescue.

Gear Depending on the remoteness and rigor of the trail, there are many additional useful items to consider: pocketknife, flashlight, fire source (waterproof matches, light, or flint), and a first-aid kit. Every member of your party should carry the appropriate essential items described above; groups often split up or get separated along the trail. Solo hikers should be even more disciplined about preparation, and carry more gear. Traveling solo is inherently more risky. This isn't meant to discourage solo travel, simply to emphasize the need for extra preparation.

Trail Etiquette

The overriding rule on the trail is **"Leave No Trace."** Interest in visiting natural areas continues to increase in North America, even as the quantity of unspoiled natural areas continues to shrink. These pressures make it ever more critical that we leave no trace of our visits.

Never Litter If you carried it in, it's easy enough to carry it out. Leave the trail in the same, if not better condition than you find it. Try picking up any litter you encounter and packing it out—it's a great feeling! Pick up just one piece of garbage and you've made a difference.

Stay on the Trail Paths have been created, sometimes over many years, for many purposes: to protect the surrounding natural areas, to avoid dangers, and to provide the best route. Leaving the trail can cause damage that takes years to undo. Never cut switchbacks. Shortcutting rarely saves energy or time, and it takes a terrible toll on the land, trampling plant life and hastening erosion. Moreover, safety and consideration intersect on the trail. It's hard to get truly lost if you stay on the trail.

Share the Trail The best trails attract many visitors, and you should be prepared to share the trail with others. Do your part to minimize impact.

Commonly accepted trail etiquette dictates that **bike riders yield to both hikers and equestrians, hikers yield to horseback riders, downhill hikers yield to uphill hikers, and everyone stays to the right.** Not everyone knows these rules of the road, so let commonsense and good humor be the final guide.

Leave It There   Destruction or removal of plants and animals or historical, prehistoric, or geological items is certainly unethical and almost always illegal.

Getting Lost   If you become lost on the trail, stay on the trail. Stop and take stock of the situation. In many cases, a few minutes of calm reflection will yield a solution. Consider all the clues available; use the sun to identify directions if you don't have a compass. If you determine that you are indeed lost, stay on the main trail and stay put. You are more likely to encounter other people if you stay in one place.

CHAPTER 1

Abrams Creek and Cades Cove Area

Abrams Creek and Cades Cove Area

The Abrams Creek and Cades Cove area occupies the most north-westerly parcel of the Tennessee Smokies. The section stretches from Chilhowee Mountain in the west, where the Foothills Parkway reveals overlooks aplenty to the major park entrance near the community of Townsend, where the Little River exits the park boundaries. Cades Cove, the world-famous bucolic former farming valley, is the showcase of the area. It presents a window to the agricultural past in a vale still carpeted in mountain-ringed fields. To the south stand the state line ridge and the Appalachian Trail, rising upward of 5,000 feet. Rich Mountain and other, lower ridges seal off Cades Cove from the "outside world."

Hiking trails extend like spokes from Cades Cove, accessing the entire area. Abrams Creek Ranger Station, in the far west, offers the other major trail access. This locale is the park's lowest, tucked away on a dead-end road, reaching what I believe is the world's most beautiful stream—Abrams Creek. Abrams Creek drains nearly the entire area. Trout-filled mountain rills flow off the Smokies crest and feed Abrams as it flows (sometimes underground) through Cades Cove. At the cove's western end the stream begins cutting a gorge, making a popular waterfall. It picks up other major tributaries before flowing past Abrams Creek Campground and ranger station, then enters a final wild stretch before exiting the park at Chilhowee Lake. The mouth of Abrams Creek at Chilhowee Lake is, at 875 feet, the absolute lowest point in the entire park.

Area streams have both trout and smallmouth bass. Dense rhododendron and mountain laurel thickets border the waterways while black birch, tulip trees, and other moisture-loving trees shade the valleys. Regal white pines tower over creekside flats. Pine-oak forest complexes rise on drier sites. The forests transition to northern hardwoods up high, with beech, yellow birch, and cherry rising on the ridges.

Looking west *at the Smokies crest from Rocky Top (Trail 7)*

Entering Cades Cove is a trip back in time. Several preserved log cabins and homesteads dot the valley, which at one time had extensive agricultural operations, unlike most former Smokies denizens, eking out a subsistence existence on small rocky plots. Residents drove their cattle on what's left of mountaintop meadows that still bear their names: Spence Field, Russell Field, and Gregory Bald. Logging was never widespread in the area. In fact, the upper part of the mostly trailless Panther Creek Valley, a tributary of Abrams Creek, is now a forgotten haven of a large fire-dependent pine-oak complex that barely saw an axe.

The trail system here is extensive. Cades Cove and its auto access, Laurel Creek Road, are the main jumping-off points. An 11-mile road circles Cades Cove, and not only accesses trailheads, but also is popular with windshield tourists and bicyclers. Here, hikers can head to the high country and the Appalachian Trail along the state line, or wander the lesser mountains that form the park's north boundary. Rich Mountain Road reaches but one trailhead. The Abrams Creek access, where many loop hikes are possible, offers a quiet contrast to sometimes-busy Cades Cove. Cades Cove visitors can overnight at a convenient and large campground located in the heart of the action. The 159 reservable sites are open year-round. Campers hike, rent bikes, ride horses, or fish. Abrams Creek has a smaller first-come, first-served 16-site campground, generally open from mid-March through October. More civilized accommodations can be had in nearby Townsend.

The hikes described are both loops and out-and-back treks. Along the way you can see local highlights: Abrams Falls, Gregory Bald, Spence Field, the Oliver Cabin, and good ol' Rocky Top, heralded in the nearby University of Tennessee's fight song. Other treks travel lesser trod trails, such as Pine Mountain and Turkeypen Ridge, where park beauty is subtler.

Permits

Permits are *not* required for dayhiking. Backpackers must get a backcountry permit to stay at one of the 17 designated backcountry campsites and trail shelters located in this area. Some require a simple self-registration; several require a reservation, which you can make by calling the backcountry permit office at (865) 436-1231. Pick up and fill out backcountry permits at Cades Cove Campground and Ranger Station and at a trailhead parking area kiosk near the normally unstaffed Abrams Creek Ranger Station. When you come from Townsend, you can obtain a permit at a kiosk near the gift shop at Great Smoky Mountains Institute at Tremont.

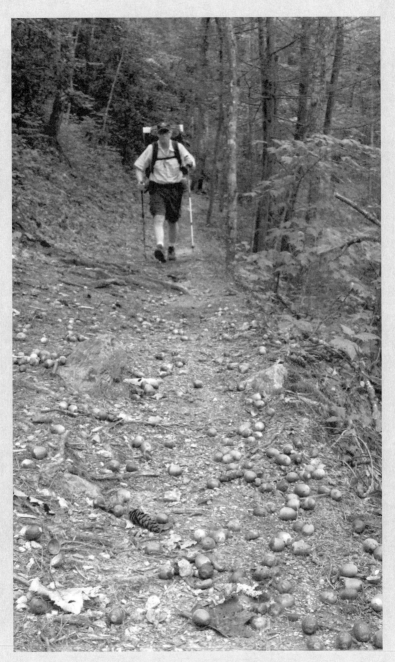

A backpacker intrepidly tackles *acorn-laden Turkeypen Ridge Trail (part of the Finley Cane Loop, Trail 8).*

Abrams Creek and Cades Cove Area

0 1 2 3 miles
0 1 2 3 kilometers

N

411

321

Little River

Chilhowee
Mountain

Maryville

Melrose

Crooked Creek

Mount
Nebo

Webb Knob

Foothills Parkway

Little
Mountain

Flat Creek

Alie
Mountain

321

Townsend

73

Laurel Lake

Foothills Parkway

Rich Mountain Road

Ellis Butt

GREAT SMOKY
MOUNTAINS
NATIONAL PARK

Cerulean
Knob

Cades Cove
Mountain

8

Cades Cove

1 2

Abrams Creek

5

7

Laurel Creek Road

6

3

Pine
Mountain

Cades Cove Loop Road

Anthony Creek

Coon Butt

Mill Creek

Parson Branch Road

4

Abrams Creek and Cades Cove Area

TRAIL	Difficulty	Length	Type	USES & ACCESS	TERRAIN	FLORA & FAUNA	OTHER
1	2–3	8.1	Loop	Dayhiking, Backpacking, Horses	Stream, Mountain, Summit	Autumn Colors, Wildflowers	Great Views, Swimming
2	3	11.0	Out & Back	Dayhiking, Backpacking	Stream, Ridgeline, Waterfall	Autumn Colors, Wildflowers	Great Views, Swimming, Photo Opportunity
3	2	5.0	Out & Back	Dayhiking	Stream, Ridgeline, Waterfall	Autumn Colors, Wildflowers	Swimming, Photo Opportunity
4	4	11.0	Out & Back	Dayhiking, Backpacking	Stream, Mountain, Summit	Autumn Colors, Wildflowers	Great Views, Photo Opportunity
5	1–2	2.8	Out & Back	Dayhiking, Backpacking, Horses, Child Friendly	Stream	Autumn Colors, Wildflowers, Wildlife	Great Views, Historic Interest, Photo Opportunity
6	4–5	13.0	Loop	Dayhiking, Backpacking, Horses	Stream, Mountain	Autumn Colors, Wildflowers	Great Views, Historic Interest
7	5	11.6	Out & Back	Dayhiking, Backpacking, Horses	Stream, Ridgeline	Autumn Colors, Wildflowers	Great Views, Photo Opportunity, Historic Interest
8	2	8.8	Loop	Dayhiking, Horses	Stream, Ridgeline	Autumn Colors, Wildflowers	Secluded, Historic Interest

USES & ACCESS
- Dayhiking
- Backpacking
- Horses
- Child Friendly

TYPE
- Loop
- Out & Back
- Point-to-Point

DIFFICULTY
- 1 2 3 4 5 +
less   more

TERRAIN
- Mountain
- Summit
- Ridgeline
- Stream
- Waterfall
- Lake

FLORA & FAUNA
- Autumn Colors
- Wildflowers
- Wildlife
- Spruce-fir
- Old-growth

FEATURES
- Great Views
- Photo Opportunity
- Backcountry Camping
- Swimming
- Secluded
- Steep
- Historic Interest
- Geologic Interest

Maps

For the Abrams Creek and Cades Cove area, you will need the following USGS 7.5-minute (1:24,000-scale) topographic quadrangles, listed in the order that you will need them as you hike along your route:

Trail 1: Calderwood
Trail 2: Calderwood
Trail 3: Cades Cove, Calderwood
Trail 4: Cades Cove
Trail 5: Cades Cove
Trail 6: Cades Cove, Thunderhead Mountain
Trail 7: Thunderhead Mountain
Trail 8: Wear Cove, Thunderhead Mountain

Abrams Creek and Cades Cove Area

TRAIL 1

Dayhiking, Horses,
Backpacking
8.1 miles, Loop
Difficulty: 1 **2** 3 4 5

Pine Mountain Loop 27
From the park's lowest trailhead, follow lovely Abrams Creek on a watery hike past numerous shoals and huge pools, eventually fording the big stream. A low ridge offers views of Look Rock. Wander through oak woods to Scott Gap, then reach a high point on the shoulder of Pine Mountain. Descend to Abrams Creek, this time spanning it by bridge.

TRAIL 2

Dayhiking, Backpacking
11.0 miles, Out & Back
Difficulty: 1 2 **3** 4 5

**Abrams Falls via Abrams Creek
Ranger Station** 33
Travel the ultrascenic and lesser visited Abrams Creek valley to reach a signature Smokies' waterfall. Much of the hike travels through the rugged Abrams Creek gorge, offering streamside views and continuous beauty. Vistas of Chilhowee Mountain open in places.

TRAIL 3

Dayhiking
5.0 miles, Out & Back
Difficulty: 1 **2** 3 4 5

Abrams Falls via Cades Cove 39
The hike to Abrams Falls from Cades Cove can be peopled, but the sight and sounds of the wide falls are an experience to be shared by one and all. The trail to the falls, alternately coursing among waterside evergreens and hillside piney woods, parallels Abrams Creek in unbroken beauty. The falls is a true rumbler and has an incredibly large pool.

Gregory Bald via Gregory Ridge 43

This classic hike takes you to a signature Smokies' destination. Follow Forge Creek past big trees in a deep valley then rise to Gregory Ridge, which leads to the state line. Take the Gregory Bald Trail to an open field with world-renowned wild azalea displays, berries in season, and a first-rate view of nearby Cades Cove, the state line ridge, and waves of mountains beyond.

TRAIL 4

Dayhiking, Backpacking
11.0 miles, Out & Back
Difficulty: 1 2 3 **4** 5

John Oliver Cabin via Rich Mountain Loop Trail 49

Walk the edge of field and forest, drinking in views of Cades Cove and the mountains that rim it. Cross a few streams then come to the historic John Oliver Cabin, built in 1820. Absorb a way of life that went on for nearly 120 years before the Smoky Mountains National Park came to be.

TRAIL 5

Dayhiking, Horses,
Child Friendly
2.8 miles, Out & Back
Difficulty: **1 2** 3 4 5

Spence Field and Russell Field Loop 55

This is a classic Smokies loop, done as either a dayhike or overnight adventure. Leave Cades Cove along scenic Anthony Creek. Rise to Bote Mountain, reaching Spence Field and the Appalachian Trail. Gain views from what is left of Spence Field. Take the AT to Russell Field trail shelter. From there, it is downhill on slender Ledbetter Ridge. Finally rejoin Anthony Creek for the return trip to Cades Cove.

TRAIL 6

Dayhiking, Horses,
Backpacking
13.0 miles, Loop
Difficulty: 1 2 3 **4 5**

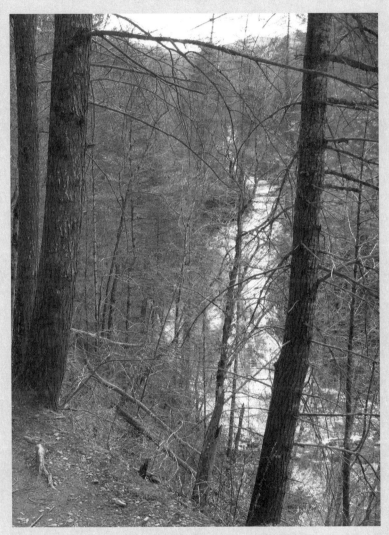

Abrams Creek *noisily rambles toward the big drop of Abrams Falls.*

Pine Mountain Loop

TRAIL 1

Bell Branch

Kingfisher Creek

Cooper Road Trail

Buck Shank Branch

Mill Branch

Hatcher Mountain Trail

Campsite #1

Little Bottoms Trail

Abrams Creek

Abrams Creek Road

Cooper Road Trail

Campsite #17

P

start & finish

Rabbit Creek Trail

To Maryville, TN

GREAT SMOKY MOUNTAINS NATIONAL PARK

Abrams Falls Trail

Abrams Creek

Hannah Mountain Trail

Pardon Branch

Pine Mountain

Rabbit Creek Trail

Rabbit Creek

Campsite #16

Hannah Mountain Trail

Campsite #15

Hannah Branch

N

0   0.2   0.4   0.6 miles

0   0.2   0.4   0.6 kilometers

Pine Mountain Loop

From the park's lowest trailhead, follow lovely Abrams Creek on a watery hike past numerous shoals and huge pools, eventually fording the big stream. A low ridge offers views of Look Rock. Wander through oak woods to Scott Gap, then reach a high point on the shoulder of Pine Mountain. Descend to Abrams Creek, this time spanning it by bridge.

Best Time

This hike requires making what is the biggest ford in the park—lower Abrams Creek. With that in mind, midsummer through late fall offers the lowest water for fording. Outside that, winter offers great solitude, and the low elevations make this hike doable when the high country is frigid. In May, the mountain laurel blooms in the Abrams Creek watershed can be spectacular.

Finding the Trail

From Maryville, Tennessee, take US 129 south, Alcoa Highway, on to Chilhowee Lake. Once at Chilhowee Lake, continue to the intersection with the Foothills Parkway. From there, keep south on US 129 for 0.5 mile farther to Happy Valley Road. Turn left on Happy Valley Road, following it 6 miles to Abrams Creek Road. Turn right on Abrams Creek Road and drive 0.7 mile, passing the ranger station. The parking area is on the right just after the ranger station. Cooper Road Trail starts at the rear of the campground.

TRAIL USE
Dayhiking, Horses,
 Backpacking

LENGTH
8.1 miles, 4–5½ hours

VERTICAL FEET
+1,000/-1,000

DIFFICULTY
− 1 **2 3** 4 5 +

TRAIL TYPE
Loop

FEATURES
Stream
Ridgeline
Summit
Autumn Colors
Wildflowers
Great Views
Swimming

FACILITIES
Water
Restrooms
Seasonal campground

Park your car in the designated area near the ranger station. *Do not park in the campground, which is gated during the cold season.*

Trail Description

This hike would be rated less difficult if it weren't for the ford of Abrams Creek, widely regarded as the most difficult in the park. But don't let the ford discourage you from taking this scenic loop hike. A drive-up campground and three backcountry campsites along the route make trailside overnighting easy. First you will leave Abrams Creek Ranger Station, tracing a gravel park road to Abrams Creek Campground. Join Cooper Road Trail, rambling along Abrams Creek to meet small Kingfisher Creek. Surmount a ridge with views to enter the rugged Abrams Creek gorge, passing Little Bottoms Campsite, #17.

Explore the park's pine-oak forested western end in a less peopled setting.

Wander through a past burn on an open rocky mountainside before reaching the potentially troublesome ford. Beyond here, it is uphill through quiet pine-oak woods to make Scott Gap. Join an old jeep road to skirt the western shoulder of Pine Mountain, presenting westerly views especially after a devastating tornado downed thousands of trees

TRAIL 1 Pine Mountain Loop Elevation Profile

A backpacker feels her way *across Abrams Creek.*

in April 2011. Descend via switchbacks on the thickly wooded north side of Pine Mountain to reach Abrams Creek yet again near old homesites. A footlog avails a safe ending to the hike.

Leave the parking area, ▶1 walking the gravel road upstream along Abrams Creek. Reach quaint 16-site Abrams Creek Campground at 0.4 mile. Pass around a pole gate, joining Cooper Road Trail ▶2 as it traverses a streamside flat over which tower tall white pines. Beech, maple, and holly are scattered in the understory. Surmount a small bluff then come to Kingfisher Branch at 0.9 mile. The trail and stream become one for a short distance then divide.

Reach a trail junction at 1.3 miles. ▶3 Cooper Road backcountry campsite, #1 is just a short ways farther on Cooper Road Trail, but this hike turns right on Little Bottoms Trail, crossing Kingfisher Branch a final time. Pass the cool waters of small Herndon Spring, located at the base of a dead hemlock, just before climbing a ridge. The 200-foot ascent leads through scrubby woodlands, recovering from fire. Look left, for northwesterly views of Chilhowee Mountain and the tower at Look Rock.

 Backcountry Camping

 Great Views

Descend from a gap in the ridge. The rumbles of Abrams Creek return. The slender single-track path winds along the gorge slope, finding Abrams Creek at 2.0 miles. Here, Buck Shank Branch—one of the Smokies all-time great names—flows into Abrams Creek. Now, you hike directly along the rock-strewn waterway, bordered by alder. Mountain laurel flanks the path.

At 2.5 miles, step over Mill Branch (a common Smokies name) and enter Little Bottoms, a now-wooded flat, once a settler home and farm. The hiking is easy here. Pass the official spur trail to Little Bottoms backcountry campsite, #17, at 2.9 miles. ▶4

The scenery changes as the gorge closes and the path rises to a steep slope, scarred by past fires and the April 2011 tornado. Open onto a rocky treeless incline with Abrams Creek crashing below. Westerly views of Chilhowee Mountain open here, too. The slender path meets Hatcher Mountain Trail at 3.6 miles. ▶5 Stay right and downhill, now on Hatcher Mountain Trail, to reach another trail junction in a streamside rhododendron thicket at 3.8 miles. ▶6 Stay right with the Hannah Mountain Trail, immediately fording Abrams Creek. Use your trekking poles or grab a stick to aid your crossing of the irregular depths. Avoid the ultraslippery flat rock slabs. In late summer or fall, the crossing will be a minor nuisance, but in winter or early spring use good judgment as to whether or not to ford.

Climb from Abrams Creek, turning up a dark rhododendron hollow. Other greenery includes galax, white pine, and holly. At 4.4 miles, split a gap. Cruise piney south-facing slopes on a nearly level needle-carpeted track. Reach clear Scott Gap Branch at 5.1 miles. Make Scott Gap and a five-way trail junction at 5.4 miles. ▶7 Backcountry campsite #16 is down the least-used path and has a small spring.

Our loop turns right on the wide, rocky double-track Rabbit Creek Trail, heading away from Rabbit

Stream

Backcountry Camping

Stream

Creek and up the shoulder of Pine Mountain, where views of the ridges and hollows of the lower Abrams Creek valley open. Dogwood, sourwood, sassafras, and pine provide colorful fall displays.

Reach the loop's high point, 2,050 feet, at 6.0 miles. ▶8 The ensuing descent off the mountain's

 Summit

north slope is mostly gentle. Here is where the tornado downed an amazing number of trees. It took months to clear the track and reopen the trail. Make hard switchbacks at 6.4 and 6.8 miles, as the wide wooded trail winds downhill. Another switchback at 7.5 miles opens a view of Abrams Creek. Soon reach the stream bottoms, passing a pair of homesites.

At 7.8 miles, bridge Abrams Creek on an ingenious footlog. ▶9 The side you are on is set on a concrete footing designed to let the footlog slide off in flood. The other side is chained to a big boulder, allowing it to turn downstream in high water yet not float away. After floods, the unchained side of the log is restored. Turn upstream beyond the crossing. Soon reach Abrams Creek Ranger Station, completing your hike at 8.1 miles. ▶10

✦	MILESTONES	
▶1	0.0	Abrams Creek parking area
▶2	0.4	Cooper Road Trail at Abrams Creek Campground
▶3	1.3	Little Bottoms Trail
▶4	2.9	Campsite #17 spur
▶5	3.6	Hatcher Mountain Trail
▶6	3.8	Hannah Mountain Trail and Abrams Creek ford
▶7	5.4	Scott Gap
▶8	6.0	Pine Mountain high point
▶9	7.8	Abrams Creek
▶10	8.1	Abrams Creek parking area

Abrams Falls via Abrams Creek Ranger Station   TRAIL 2

Cane Creek

Flat Creek

Cane Gap

Gold Mine Trail

Cane Creek Trail

GREAT SMOKY
MOUNTAINS
NATIONAL PARK

Gold
Mine
Gap

Cooper Road Trail

Kingfisher Creek

Bell Branch

Cooper Road Trail

Buck Shank Branch

Campsite #1

Little Bottoms Trail

Abrams Creek

Mill Branch

Oak Flats Branch

Beard Cane Trail

Cooper
Road Tra

Hatcher Mountain Trail

Kreider Branch

Abrams
Creek Road

Cooper Road Trail

Campsite #17

start &
finish

P

Abrams
Falls Trail

Abrams Creek

Abrams
Falls

To
Maryville, TN

Abrams Creek

Rabbit
Creek Trail

Hannah Mountain Trail

Rabbit Creek

McCully Branch

Pine
Mountain

Campsite #16

Hannah Mountain Trail

Pardon Branch

Campsite
#15

Rabbit Creek Trail

N

Hannah Mountain Trail

Hannah Branch

| 0 | 0.3 | 0.6 | 0.9 miles |
| 0 | 0.3 | 0.6 | 0.9 kilometers |

Abrams Falls via Abrams Creek Ranger Station

Travel the ultrascenic and lesser visited Abrams Creek valley to reach a signature Smokies' waterfall. Much of the hike travels through the rugged Abrams Creek gorge, offering streamside views and continuous beauty. Vistas of Chilhowee Mountain open in places.

Best Time

Abrams Falls will be its boldest during winter and spring. You will also enjoy solitude and relatively mild winter temperatures on this lowland trek that never rises above 1,600 feet of elevation. May has the added benefit of trailside mountain laurel blooms. Summer brings crowds to the falls, the vast majority coming from Cades Cove.

Finding the Trail

From Maryville, Tennessee, take US 129 south, Alcoa Highway, on to Chilhowee Lake. Once at Chilhowee Lake, continue to the intersection with the Foothills Parkway. From there, keep south on US 129 for 0.5 mile farther to Happy Valley Road. Turn left on Happy Valley Road, following it 6 miles to Abrams Creek Road. Turn right on Abrams Creek Road and drive 0.7 mile, passing the ranger station.

The parking area is on the right just after the ranger station. Cooper Road Trail starts at the rear of the campground. Park your car in the designated area near the ranger station. *Do not park in the campground, which is gated during the cold season.*

TRAIL USE
Dayhiking, Backpacking

LENGTH
11.0 miles, 6 hours

VERTICAL FEET
+500/-500

DIFFICULTY
− 1 2 **3** 4 5 +

TRAIL TYPE
Out & Back

FEATURES
Stream
Ridgeline
Waterfall
Autumn Colors
Wildflowers
Great Views
Swimming
Photo Opportunity

SEASONAL FACILITIES
Water
Restrooms
Campground

Trail Description

This great hike explores lower Abrams Creek, including a visit to a powerful cataract, coupled with hillside views. While Abrams Falls is a popular destination, you will be taking the back way. It is longer but avails much more solitude. The hills are ample enough to challenge but not overwhelm you. Since the hike starts near a drive-up campground and you pass two backcountry campsites along the way, combining an overnight experience with this hike is easy.

Your return trip is sure to add new sights. Make sure and stop along the way to absorb some Abrams Creek streamside scenery. You will have plenty of opportunities since the trail is near the creek at multiple junctures.

Leave the parking area, ▶1 walking the gravel road upstream along Abrams Creek. Anglers and swimmers wanting easy access will be seen here in the summer. Curve right to reach Abrams Creek Campground. The 16 sites are situated in a teardrop loop. Campers coming during the week are sure to get a site.

At 0.4 mile, walk around a pole gate, joining the Cooper Road Trail. ▶2 A regal forest of white pines

TRAIL 2 Abrams Falls via Abrams Creek Ranger Station Elevation Profile

shades smaller beech, maple, and holly. The path rises to a small bluff. Abrams Creek gurgles at the bluff base. Descend to Kingfisher Branch at 0.9 mile. The trail and stream merge. You are sure to do a little rock-hopping here, depending on water levels.

Stream

Meet the Little Bottoms Trail at 1.3 miles. ▶3 Cooper Road backcountry campsite, #1, is about 50 yards beyond on Cooper Road Trail. However, the hike to Abrams Falls turns right and joins the Little Bottoms Trail. Immediately, rock-hop Kingfisher Branch.

Backcountry Camping

As you continue, look for small Herndon Spring, located at the base of a dead hemlock, just before the Little Bottoms starts to scale a ridge dividing Kingfisher Creek from Abrams Creek. Switchbacks moderate the 200-foot ascent. Walk among scrubby young trees, regenerating after the Buck Shank Fire of 2007. The bushy trees allow northwesterly views of Chilhowee Mountain and the tower at Look Rock.

Great Views

Descend from a gap in the ridge. Abrams Creek bellows below. The slender single-track path winds along the gorge slope, descending to the mouth of Buck Shank Branch. This stream lent its interesting name to the fire, more of which you will walk through. Alder and mountain laurel border the trail, running directly beside Abrams Creek.

Stream

At 2.5 miles, hop over Mill Branch and reach Little Bottoms, a now-wooded flat isolated within the Abrams Creek gorge. An isolation-seeking settler once called this home. Imagine these woods being a tilled field. Curve around Little Bottoms. Spur paths lead left to Little Bottoms backcountry campsite, #17, but you reach the official spur trail (with a signpost) at 2.9 miles. ▶4

Wildflowers

Backcountry Camping

The gorge closes and the trail angles onto a steep open slope laid bare after an incredible and rare 2011 tornado. Cruise along an open rock outcrop dropping sharply below. Look back, westerly, to see the ridge of Chilhowee Mountain. The slender

If you are unwilling to walk 5 miles one-way to worthy Abrams Falls, consider coming from Cades Cove.

path meets Hatcher Mountain Trail at 3.6 miles. Stay right and downhill, joining Hatcher Mountain Trail. ►5 Reach a trail junction in rhododendron at 3.8 miles. Here, the Hannah Mountain Trail leaves right to ford Abrams Creek and makes for a good streamside relaxing spot.

Stay left, joining the Abrams Falls Trail, ►6 a little tamer than Little Bottoms Trail. Tunnel through thick woods and rhododendron. Abrams Creek is a little smaller. You are now upstream of its confluence with major tributary Rabbit Creek. The trail turns northeast, mimicking the wanderings

A hiker poses *in front of crashing Abrams Falls.*

of Abrams Creek. The foot trail is simply gorgeous here. Rise to meet Oak Flats Branch at 4.3 miles. ▶7 The path soon bisects Kreider Branch. The trail then climbs a dry slope well above the creek. Gain top-down views of singing rapids below. The creek turns away. The trail is bisecting a bend in the creek.

Level off at 5.1 miles, ▶8 at the hike's high point of 1,550 feet, then cruise downhill to reach a trail junction at 5.5 miles. Here, a spur trail leads straight over a footlog spanning Wilson Branch while the Abrams Falls Trail leaves left for Cades Cove.

Beyond the bridge, you come to the massive pool below powerful Abrams Falls. Sitting rocks and logs abound. Abrams Falls roars in the distance. Walk to the base of the potent cataract. ▶9 The powerful cascade drops 20 feet over a rock berm.

In summer you may be surprised at the throngs that have walked 2.5 miles from Cades Cove, while so few have hiked your route. The pool is one of the park's deepest and lures sweaty hikers trekking in the summer heat. Hopefully, you have enough time to linger at the falls and stop a time or two on your way back as well. Abrams Creek is my favorite waterway in the entire park.

> **The Buck Shank Fire, believed to be caused by humans, burned around 1,000 acres before the park service contained it.**

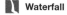 **Waterfall**

		MILESTONES
▶1	0.0	Abrams Creek parking area
▶2	0.4	Cooper Road Trail at Abrams Creek Campground
▶3	1.3	Little Bottoms Trail
▶4	2.9	Campsite #17 spur
▶5	3.6	Hatcher Mountain Trail
▶6	3.8	Join Abrams Falls Trail
▶7	4.3	Oak Flats Branch
▶8	5.1	Hike high point
▶9	5.5	Abrams Falls

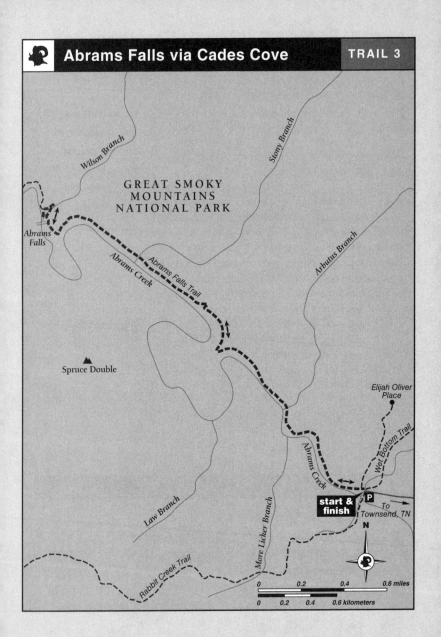

Abrams Falls via Cades Cove
TRAIL 3

GREAT SMOKY
MOUNTAINS
NATIONAL PARK

Wilson Branch

Stony Branch

Arbutus Branch

Abrams
Falls

Abrams Falls Trail

Abrams Creek

Spruce Double

Elijah Oliver
Place

Wet Bottom Trail

Abrams Creek

start &
finish

P

To
Townsend, TN

N

Law Branch

More Licker Branch

Rabbit Creek Trail

| 0 | 0.2 | 0.4 | 0.6 miles |

| 0 | 0.2 | 0.4 | 0.6 kilometers |

Abrams Falls via Cades Cove

The hike to Abrams Falls from Cades Cove can be peopled, but the sight and sounds of the wide falls are an experience to be shared by one and all. The trail to the falls, alternately coursing among waterside evergreens and hillside piney woods, parallels Abrams Creek in unbroken beauty. The falls is a true rumbler and has an incredibly large pool.

Best Time

Winter offers the most solitude. The falls will be their boldest then and in spring. Summer can be hot and crowded but is good for swimming. Consider going early or late in the day during potentially busy times.

Finding the Trail

From Townsend, Tennessee, take TN 73 to enter the park at the Townsend Wye. Turn right on Laurel Creek Road and follow it for 7.4 miles to the beginning of Cades Cove Loop Road. Join one-way Cades Cove Loop Road for 5.1 miles, then turn right on the marked spur road for 0.4 mile to the Abrams Falls Trailhead.

Trail Description

The parking area can be busy and the trailhead can be confusing. ▶1 First-time hikers to Abrams Falls can often surreptitiously follow others onto the correct path. You will see the Rabbit Creek Trail leaving left for Hannah Mountain. The Abrams Falls Trail

TRAIL USE
Dayhiking
LENGTH
5.0 miles, 2½–3 hours
VERTICAL FEET
+300/-300
DIFFICULTY
– 1 **2** 3 4 5 +
TRAIL TYPE
Out & Back

FEATURES
Stream
Ridgeline
Waterfall
Autumn Colors
Wildflowers
Swimming
Photo Opportunity

FACILITIES
None

Stream

Autumn Colors

Wildflowers

Ridgeline

From Arbutus Ridge
you can see Abrams
Creek coming and
going as it works
around the horseshoe.

goes straight, bridging Abrams Creek while the Wet
Bottom Trail leaves right for Cooper Road Trail. Take
the Abrams Falls Trail over Abrams Creek. Here, a
trail leaves right; take it and in a half mile reach the
Elijah Oliver Place, a potential historical addition
to your trek. Ahead, you can see the inflow of Mill
Creek, which significantly adds to Abrams Creek.

Begin tracing the crashing creek downstream.
Shortly climb above the greenish watercourse,
under pine, beech, birch, and oak. Rhododendron
and mountain laurel border the track. Spur trails
lead to the water. Be careful if you head to the creek,
the rocks underwater are notoriously slick! Bridge
Arbutus Branch on a footlog at 0.6 mile. ▶2 A favorable water access is just beyond the .

At 1.1 miles, after ascending a slaty hill on a
rocky tread, the trail crosses Arbutus Ridge. ▶3
Meanwhile, Abrams Creek is working around the
ridge, forming a horseshoe. Descend to Abrams
Creek, crossing a creeklet at 1.4 miles. Alternately
travel creekside and farther up the ridgeside to
view the watercourse from different perspectives
as well as work your muscles a bit. At 1.8 miles,
cross Stony Branch on a footlog. ▶4 You may see
the blackened bases of trailside tree trunks. This is
part of the greater Buck Shank Fire. Climb another
hill and at 2.3 miles you can hear and partially see

TRAIL 3 Abrams Falls via Cades Cove Elevation Profile

Even deer *enjoy hiking to Abrams Falls via Cades Cove.*

Abrams Falls. Descend to Wilson Branch, bridging it by footlog before returning to Abrams Creek. Cross back over Wilson Branch on another footlog and you are there. ►5

The wide plunge pool below the falls is nearly as impressive as the falls itself. Note the log jumble at the lower end of the pool. In the summer the pool is a popular swimming hole. The falls themselves, wide and powerful, descend in a roar of power and mist, quite a sight.

Waterfall

 Swimming

🚶	**MILESTONES**	
►1	0.0	Cades Cove Loop Road Trailhead
►2	0.6	Cross Arbutus Branch
►3	1.1	Arbutus Ridge
►4	1.8	Bridge Stony Branch
►5	2.5	Abrams Falls

Gregory Bald via Gregory Ridge

TRAIL 4

Rabbit Creek

Coalen Ground Branch

Forge Creek Road

P

To Townsend, TN

start & finish

Forge Creek

Tiptons Sugar Cove

Tiptons Sugar Cove Branch

Sugar Cove Ridge

GREAT SMOKY MOUNTAINS NATIONAL PARK

Campsite #12

Bower Creek

Gregory Ridge Trail

Gregory Ridge

Forge Creek

Brier Lick Branch

High Point

N

Gregory Bald Trail

Gregory Bald Trail

Campsite #13

Gregory Bald

Gregory Little Bald

Long Hungry Ridge Trail

| 0 | 0.2 | 0.4 | 0.6 miles |
| 0 | 0.2 | 0.4 | 0.6 kilometers |

Gregory Bald via Gregory Ridge

This classic hike takes you to a signature Smokies' destination. Follow Forge Creek past big trees in a deep valley then rise to Gregory Ridge, which leads to the state line. Take the Gregory Bald Trail to an open field with world-renowned wild azalea displays, berries in season, and a first-rate view of nearby Cades Cove, the state line ridge, and waves of mountains beyond.

Best Time

Hike the trail in spring for streamside wildflowers and good views. June can be hazy but that's when the world-famous wild azaleas bloom. Come in July and early August for blueberries. Views once again become far-reaching when fall cold fronts clear the skies. Winter can be very windy and cold atop the open parts of Gregory Bald.

Finding the Trail

From Townsend, Tennessee, follow Laurel Creek Road to Cades Cove. Join and follow Cades Cove Loop Road for 5.5 miles, then turn right on Forge Creek Road. This intersection is near the Cable Mill visitor center. Follow Forge Creek Road for 2.3 miles to the turnaround and the Gregory Ridge Trail.

Trail Description

This hike is packed with features to satisfy even the most demanding hiker. On the way to Gregory Bald pass a mountain stream bordered by old-growth

TRAIL USE
Dayhiking, Backpacking

LENGTH
11.0 miles,
5½–7½ hours

VERTICAL FEET
+2,980/-2,980

DIFFICULTY
– 1 2 3 **4** 5 +

TRAIL TYPE
Out & Back

FEATURES
Stream
Ridgeline
Summit
Autumn Colors
Wildflowers
Great Views
Photo Opportunity

FACILITIES
Camping
Restrooms at nearby
Cable Mill visitor
center

woodland, and ascend a ridge. Take a side trip to historic Moore Spring, where an Appalachian Trail shelter once stood. It's a steady climb to the bald, but well worth it.

Make a short, quick ascent in pines upon leaving Forge Creek Road, ▶1 to join up with Forge Creek proper, crossing it on a footbridge at 0.3 mile. ▶2 A little less a mile into the hike, large tulip trees rise tall above the mountain scenery, along with smaller red maples, black birch, and rhododendron. Forge Creek gathers in pools then dashes downstream amid rocks. Climb well above the creek onto a slope above the stream. At 1.5 miles, Ekaneetlee Branch spills into Forge Creek. A historic Indian Trail once crossed the mountains at Ekaneetlee Gap then followed Ekaneetlee Branch to the confluence below. Head deeper into Forge Creek Valley. Footlogs help you cross a much smaller Forge Creek at 1.8 and 1.9 miles. ▶3 Just beyond the last crossing is the Forge Creek backcountry campsite, #12. ▶4 It is located on a hardwood knoll. Forge Creek makes a semicircle below. Fill up with water here as the rest of the way is dry until the state line.

Leave the valley behind, working up the east slope of Gregory Ridge, flanked by galax. Cut into a hollow at 2.3 miles, then emerge on a fire-scarred ridge with standing bleached tree skeletons tower-

 Stream

Wildflowers

Backcountry Camping

TRAIL 4 Gregory Bald via Gregory Ridge Elevation Profile

ing over mountain laurel and young pines. The trail twists among exposed boulders. Look right, north, for views of Cades Cove below. ►5

At 2.5 miles, the path turns south, aiming for the state line, now in a drier forest of chestnut oak, pine, and blueberries. You've worked hard to get here but the ridge keeps on rising until 3.1 miles, where the trail levels off at 3,400 feet. Grab a breather for 0.1 mile while tunneling through mountain laurel.

▲ **Ridgeline**

Slip over to the northwest side of Gregory Ridge, regaining the crest at 3.8 miles. In this upper section the path stays off the center of the ridge, away from the now-overgrown, but still rutted cattle path that once connected the state line balds to Cades Cove farms below. In pre-park days farmers drove the cattle to the balds for the summer, while they grew hay for winter in the fields below.

Looking down *on a prescribed fire in Cades Cove from Gregory Bald*

Once 15 acres, by the mid-1980s Gregory Bald was less than half that. The park service returned it to the dimension it was when grazing kept the forest from overtaking the grasses.

 Ridgeline

 Summit

Break the 4,000-foot-elevation mark at 4.0 miles. Yellow birch trees become common in this chillier clime. At 4.7 miles, the trail slips over to the southeast side of the Gregory Ridge. Winter views of the Smokies crest open, keeping your spirits high. Saunter into Rich Gap and a trail junction, at mile 4.9. The Gregory Ridge Trail ends here. ▶6 To the left 0.1 mile, the Long Hungry Ridge Trail terminates from Twentymile Ranger Station. An unmarked path leads 0.3 mile straight ahead to Moore Spring, where an Appalachian Trail shelter once stood before the AT was rerouted over Fontana Dam in the 1940s. The spring, in a small clearing, is one of the Smokies' finest.

Turn right up the Gregory Bald Trail. Ascend into beech and yellow birch rising above a rock and grass understory. Level off at 5.2 miles, then rise again, opening onto the bald. Note the wind-sculpted blueberry and azalea bushes where grasses are absent. Crest out on a field at 5.5 miles. ▶7 Note the USGS survey markers.

Flame azalea bushes bloom in an eye-popping display of oranges and reds during June. A hungry hiker can sample the blueberries later in summer. Inclement weather excepted, Gregory Bald offers nearly a 360-degree view year-round. To the south are wave upon wave of mountains of the Nantahala National Forest. The crest of the Smokies rolls away to the east. To the north, the fields of Cades Cove lie below, with East Tennessee stretching to the horizon. Sheep Pen Gap backcountry campsite, #13, lays a half mile beyond the bald on the Gregory Bald Trail.

🚶 MILESTONES

▶1   0.0   Forge Creek Trailhead

▶2   0.3   Bridge Forge Creek

▶3   1.8   Bridge Forge Creek twice in short succession

▶4   1.9   Forge Creek Campsite, #12

▶5   2.5   Gain crest of Gregory Ridge

▶6   4.9   At Rich Gap turn right on Gregory Bald Trail

▶7   5.5   Top of Gregory Bald

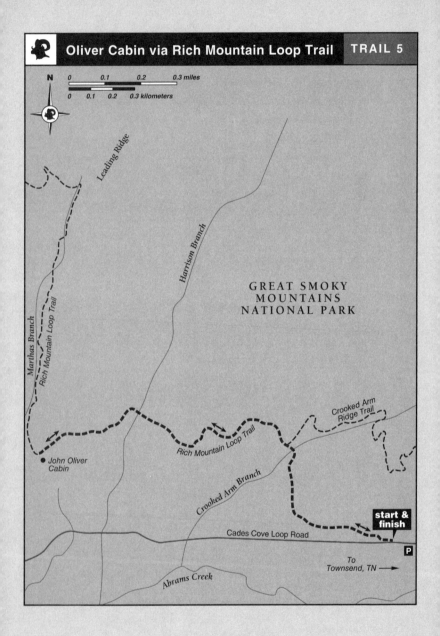

Oliver Cabin via Rich Mountain Loop Trail   TRAIL 5

N

0   0.1   0.2   0.3 miles
0   0.1   0.2   0.3 kilometers

Leading Ridge

Harrison Branch

GREAT SMOKY
MOUNTAINS
NATIONAL PARK

Marthas Branch

Rich Mountain Loop Trail

Crooked Arm
Ridge Trail

Rich Mountain Loop Trail

John Oliver
Cabin

Crooked Arm Branch

start &
finish

Cades Cove Loop Road

P

To
Townsend, TN →

Abrams Creek

John Oliver Cabin via Rich Mountain Loop Trail

Walk the edge of field and forest, drinking in views of Cades Cove and the mountains that rim it. Cross a few streams then come to the historic John Oliver Cabin, built in 1820. Absorb a way of life that went on for nearly 120 years before the Smoky Mountains National Park came to be.

Best Time

Fall through spring are the best times to make this walk. In fall, the clear skies will allow for mountain and field panoramas. Also, you may spot deer then, too. Winter will offer solitude, and since it is a low-elevation hike, it will have better weather than the high country. In spring, the stream crossings may be a little high but shouldn't pose a problem under normal conditions.

Finding the Trail

From Townsend, Tennessee, take TN 73 to enter the park at the Townsend Wye. Turn right on Laurel Creek Road and follow it for 7.4 miles to the beginning of Cades Cove Loop Road. Park at the loop's beginning in the large parking area on the left.

To pick up the Rich Mountain Loop Trail walk a short distance down the loop road, past the pole gate, to where the signed trail begins on your right. *Do not drive into one-way Cades Cove Loop Road* lest you be forced to make the entire loop or shortcut on Sparks Lane.

TRAIL USE
Dayhiking, Horses,
    Child Friendly
LENGTH
2.8 miles, 1½–2 hours
VERTICAL FEET
+90/-90
DIFFICULTY
– **1 2** 3 4 5 +
TRAIL TYPE
Out & Back

FEATURES
Stream
Autumn Colors
Wildflowers
Wildlife
Great Views
Historic Interest
Photo Opportunity

FACILITIES
Picnic area
Campground
Water
Restrooms
Camp store (seasonal)

Trail Description

In the early 1800s, Cades Cove was wildland belonging to the Cherokees. However, a treaty in 1819 opened this mountain-rimmed valley to settlement. It wasn't long after—and maybe even before 1819—when John Oliver settled in Cades Cove. Oliver had migrated south from northeast Tennessee, up Elizabethton way, where settlers were already pouring over the mountains. The former soldier, who had fought under fellow Tennessean Andrew Jackson, decided to stay a spell here in the shadow of the Smokies.

Their simple agrarian way of life seems idyllic compared to the daily rush we face today. It was a time when families worked together, following the seasons to reap what they had sown, whether it be corn (the staple of the people of Cades Cove), butchering a pig when the first frost lay down, gathering wild blueberries and blackberries from the land, or harvesting apples from planted orchards.

Today slow yourself down and take the stroll along the foot of Rich Mountain. Gain views of the state line crest that loomed over Oliver and his fellow Cades Cove residents. In the foreground, enjoy the fields of Cades Cove. They are still kept open today, preserving this pastoral backwater. And when you

TRAIL 5 Oliver Cabin via Rich Mountain Loop Elevation Profile

This cabin *was one of the first homesteads in Cades Cove.*

reach the cabin of John Oliver, walk around inside, and imagine yourself in his shoes, two centuries ago carving out a homestead and raising a family in a land that was to become a national park. It is these historic cabins that give a tangible link to a past way of life that has left us forever.

From the parking area at the beginning of Cades Cove Loop Road, ▶1 walk the loop road a short piece to join the Rich Mountain Loop Trail, a single-track dirt-and-rock path leaving right. Cades Cove Loop Road is to your left and Crooked Arm Ridge rises to your right. White pines, oaks, and tulip trees **Great Views** shade the nearly level path. By 0.3 mile, fields open to your left through tall trees that lined the former settler road. ▶2 Gain bucolic views through the trees of waving grasses with wooded mountains beyond, perhaps deer foraging in the fields. At 0.5 mile, rock-hop over seasonal Crooked Arm Branch, then come to a trail junction. ▶3

Stream

Here, the Crooked Arm Ridge Trail leaves right. Stay straight with the Rich Mountain Loop Trail as it rolls through slightly hilly wooded terrain heavy with shortleaf pines, indicating this was likely pasture or cropland in Cades Cove's heyday. Cross a small, unnamed rocky branch at 0.8 mile. ▶4 Keep a westerly course amid more pines and sourwood. At 1.0 mile, step over Harrison Branch, which can be completely dry in late summer or fall. ▶5

Stream

Wander more foothills then drift into a clearing and the John Oliver Cabin at 1.4 miles. ▶6 One legend has it that Oliver wandered into Cades Cove

A backpacker treks *past the John Oliver Cabin in the rain.*

while hunting and then spent the night in an Indian hut. Since he found the area already beautiful and potentially productive, he built his home here. This is but one of many impressive log cabins within the cove. They serve as a link to East Tennessee's rural past. John Oliver and his offspring populated the cove and never left.

Other visitors will be accessing the cabin from Cades Cove Loop Road. If bicycling, be apprised the loop road is closed to autos on Wednesday and Saturday mornings until 10 a.m. during the warm season. Camp at Cades Cove Campground, and enjoy an early start! Another option is to pedal the road under a full moon. Leave a little while before dusk and enjoy sunset and moonrise. You are required to have a flashlight if pedaling at night.

Explore the rest of Cades Cove: via the many hiking trails that lace the cove perimeter, by bicycling the 10-mile loop road, or by driving the cove loop road.

🚶	**MILESTONES**	
►1	0.0	Cades Cove Loop Road Trailhead
►2	0.3	Views of Cades Cove and beyond
►3	0.5	Crooked Arm Ridge Trail
►4	0.8	Unnamed branch
►5	1.0	Harrison Branch
►6	1.4	John Oliver Cabin

Spence Field & Russell Field Loop

TRAIL 6

To Townsend, TN

Laurel Creek

Laurel Creek Road

start & finish

P

Crib Gap Trail

Lead Cove Trail

Abrams Creek

horse camp

Cooper Branch

Laurel Cove Creek

Sugar Cove Prong

Maynard Creek

Anthony Creek Trail

Allnight Ridge

GREAT SMOKY MOUNTAINS NATIONAL PARK

Anthony Creek

Cold Water Knob

West Prong Little River

Bote Mountain Trail

Rowans Creek

Leadbetter Ridge

Campsite #10

Ledbetter Ridge Trail

Campsite #9

Left Prong Anthony Creek

Anthony Ridge

Russell Field Branch

McCampbell Knob

Maple Sugar Gap

Mount Squires

Spence Field

Russell Field Shelter

Russell Field

Spence Field Shelter

Eagle Creek Trail

Eagle Creek

N

| 0 | 0.2 | 0.4 | 0.6 miles |
| 0 | 0.2 | 0.4 | 0.6 kilometers |

Spence Field and Russell Field Loop

First day hike

This is a classic Smokies loop, done as either a dayhike or overnight adventure.. Leave Cades Cove along scenic Anthony Creek. Rise to Bote Mountain, reaching Spence Field and the Appalachian Trail. Gain views from what is left of Spence Field. Take the AT to Russell Field trail shelter. From there, it is downhill on slender Ledbetter Ridge. Finally rejoin Anthony Creek for the return trip to Cades Cove.

Best Time

Cool off during summer along Anthony Creek, then get breezes while in the high country. Fall and spring offer better views in addition to colorful foliage and wildflowers.

Finding the Trail

From Townsend, take Laurel Creek Road to Cades Cove. Just before the beginning of the Cades Cove Loop Road, turn left toward Cades Cove Campground, then immediately turn left into the picnic area. The Anthony Creek Trail is on your right at the back of the picnic area. Parking can be limited in the picnic area.

If you are backpacking be apprised *overnight parking is prohibited* in the picnic area. Instead, park in the long parking strip at the beginning of Cades Cove Loop Road or return toward the campground and park in the lot beside the campground office and camp store.

TRAIL USE
Dayhiking, Horses,
    Backpacking
LENGTH
13.0 miles, 6–8 hours
VERTICAL FEET
+3,040/-3,040
DIFFICULTY
- 1 2 3 **4 5** +
TRAIL TYPE
Loop

FEATURES
Ridgeline
Stream
Summit
Autumn Colors
Wildflowers
Great Views
Photo Opportunity
Historic Interest

FACILITIES
Campground
Picnic tables
Restrooms near
    trailhead

Trail Description

This strenuous all-day hike or satisfying overnight backpack provides ample reward to those who want to see the Smokies from bottom to top. Starting in Cades Cove, you will climb along a deeply forested, crashing mountain stream. Intersect the famed Appalachian Trail at the Smokies crest. Once on the AT, outstanding views open at Spence Field. Return to Cades Cove via Russell Field Trail with its section of old-growth trees. You pass four backcountry camping options along the way.

Pick up the double-track Anthony Creek Trail, ▶1 leaving the picnic area in preserved hemlock, tulip trees, sycamore, and rhododendron. Upper Abrams Creek crashes to your right. At 0.2 mile, the Crib Gap Trail leaves left for Turkeypen Ridge. ▶2 Continue straight and dip to pass through Anthony Creek Horse Camp. ▶3 The trail narrows beyond the camp. Bridge Abrams Creek at 0.6 mile in a once settled area. Look for leveled areas and old roadbeds.

 Stream

At 0.9 mile, span Abrams Creek on a footlog. Bridge it again at 1.1 miles. Note the rock walls on trail right at 1.4 miles, indicating another settled area, now returned to the bears. Bridge Left Prong Anthony

TRAIL 6 Spence Field & Russell Field Loop Elevation Profile

Creek at 1.6 miles then come to a trail junction. Stay left with the Anthony Creek Trail. Ledbetter Ridge Trail leaves right and is your return route. ▶4

Watch for an old chimney on your left at 1.7 miles. At 2.0 miles, bridge Anthony Creek. Keep ascending on a rocky tread. Tulip trees comprise a significant part of a majestic hardwood forest towering overhead. At 2.6 miles, step over a tributary of Anthony Creek. Continuing to climb, the trail passes the Anthony Creek backcountry campsite, #9, on your right, at 2.8 miles. ▶5 It is set in a series of somewhat tiered flats. Turn away from the campsite, leaving Anthony Creek for Bote Mountain, rising in viney cove hardwoods nestled on a north-facing slope. Wintertime views of Cades Cove open below.

Intersect Bote Mountain Trail at 3.5 miles. ▶6 Turn right on the former Cherokee-built toll road. When building the turnpike from the lowlands to the Smokies crest, the Cherokee chose the route that should be taken, "voting" for this ridge, which ended up being called "Bote Mountain," since the natives had a hard time with the letter "v." The next ridge east, not chosen, became known as Defeat Ridge.

Herders later used the wide track to drive their cattle to Spence Field for the summer. Reach an old jeep turnaround at 3.8 miles. This is where the trail narrows and becomes a deeply rutted, rocky path, bordered by moss, galax, and rhododendron. Occasional brief level sections allow a breather. Watch for a hollowed-out rock on the right at 4.6 miles. Settlers would set out salt licks for their cattle using hollowed rocks or logs. The path can be rocky or muddy. Step over a spring branch, then make your final assault on Spence Field using switchbacks that take you through buckeye, beech, and yellow birch forest. Pass a piped spring at 5.0 miles. A final

🏠 **Historic Interest**

⚠ **Backcountry Camping**

As you climb Spence Field look back for views of Thunderhead Mountain and *the Rocky Top* that inspired the UT Volunteers signature fight song.

push takes you up to the lower reaches of Spence Field and the Appalachian Trail at 5.2 miles. ▶7

Take time to explore this former pasture that still has broken fields, continually shrinking as tree cover advances. It is an ideal spot to have a snack and rest before you turn west on the Appalachian Trail toward Russell Field. Before leaving Spence Field, the AT passes the Eagle Creek Trail, where a backcountry shelter and spring are located 0.2 mile distant. Leave what is left of Spence Field and reenter beech woods. Dip to a gap at 5.6 miles, then skirt around the north side of Mount Squires. Reach the high point of your hike, breaking the 5,000-foot mark at 5.9 miles. ▶8 It is mostly downhill from here.

Slip over to the south side of the state line ridge, passing through sporadic rhododendron thickets amid hardwoods. Wintertime views into the Tar Heel State open. Step over a spring branch at 6.6 miles. Pass through Maple Sugar Gap at 7.0 miles, ▶9 and continue a downgrade. A pair of switchbacks at 7.3 miles takes you lower still. Reach McCampbell Gap at 7.7 miles, ▶10 then make a brief ascent around McCampbell Knob.

At 8.0 miles, reach Russell Field Shelter, ▶11 a trail junction and your departure from the AT. Turn right, northbound on the Russell Field Trail. Pass an evergreen-bordered spring, the headwaters of Russell Field Branch, before coming beside Russell Field at 8.4 miles. Spur trails lead right to a small relic meadow bordered by white pines.

Descend a north-facing slope, joining slender Ledbetter Ridge at 8.9 miles. The path runs nearly level in pines, oaks, mountain laurel, and maples. Make a sharp turn at 9.7 miles, ▶12 descending for a tributary of Left Prong Anthony Creek. Between the ridge and Ledbetter Ridge backcountry campsite, #10, at mile 10.6, ▶13 look for sizeable tulip trees.

Great Views

Backcountry Camping

Summit

Backcountry Camping

Backcountry Camping

The Ledbetter Ridge Trail crosses the tributary just below the campsite.

Span Left Prong Anthony Creek on a footbridge at 10.8 miles. At 11.4 miles, come again to the Anthony Creek Trail, completing the loop portion of the hike. ▶14 Retrace your steps down the Anthony Creek Trail to arrive at the Cades Cove picnic area at 13.0 miles. ▶15

🚶	**MILESTONES**

▶1	0.0	Anthony Creek Trailhead at Cades Cove Picnic Area
▶2	0.2	Crib Gap Trail leaves left
▶3	0.3	Anthony Creek Horse Camp
▶4	1.6	Ledbetter Ridge Trail leaves left
▶5	2.8	Anthony Creek backcountry campsite, #9
▶6	3.5	Right on Bote Mountain Trail
▶7	5.2	At Spence Field, turn right on Appalachian Trail
▶8	5.9	Mount Squires
▶9	7.0	Maple Sugar Gap
▶10	7.7	McCampbell Gap
▶11	8.0	At Russell Field Shelter, turn right on Ledbetter Ridge Trail
▶12	9.7	Leave Ledbetter Ridge
▶13	10.6	Ledbetter Ridge backcountry campsite, #10
▶14	11.4	Left on Anthony Creek Trail, and backtrack
▶15	13.0	Anthony Creek Trailhead at Cades Cove Picnic Area

Rocky Top via Lead Cove

TRAIL 7

start & finish

Bote Mountain ▲

Hickory Tree Branch

Laurel Creek Road

To Townsend, TN

Lead Cove Trail

Laurel Cove Creek

Sugar Cove Prong

Bote Mountain Trail

West Prong Little River

N

0   0.2   0.4   0.6 miles

0   0.2   0.4   0.6 kilometers

Sandy Gap

Devils Nest Creek

Allnight Ridge

Anthony Creek Trail

Cold Water Knob

Long Cove Creek

Anthony Creek

Bee Cove Creek

West Prong Little River

GREAT SMOKY
MOUNTAINS
NATIONAL PARK

Bote Mountain Trail

Thunderhead Mountain ▲

Rocky Top ▲

Mount Squires ▲

Spence Field

Spence Field Shelter

Eagle Creek Trail

Eagle Creek

Jenkins Ridge Trail

Rocky Top via Lead Cove

This hike is the epitome of the old adage, "You reap what you sow." You will burn a lot of calories on this climb with views as good as they come. Travel Lead Cove to intersect Bote Mountain Trail. Join the Appalachian Trail, passing through Spence Field, climbing farther still to the storied Rocky Top.

TRAIL USE
Dayhiking, Horses,
    Backpacking
LENGTH
11.6 miles, 6–8 hours
VERTICAL FEET
+3,500/-3,500
DIFFICULTY
– 1 2 3 4 **5** +
TRAIL TYPE
Out & Back

Best Time

This hike covers a lot of ecological zones as it climbs and therefore offers year-round beauty. Practically speaking, the warmer season will avail snow-free conditions up high. Fall and spring will have clear skies and the best vistas.

FEATURES
Ridgeline
Stream
Autumn Colors
Wildflowers
Great Views
Photo Opportunity
Historic Interest

Finding the Trail

From Townsend, Tennessee, drive 5.6 miles from the Townsend Wye right on Laurel Creek Road toward Cades Cove. The Lead Cove Trail is on your left just beyond a small parking area that extends on both sides of the road.

FACILITIES
Camping

Trail Description

Leave Laurel Creek Road behind ▶1 and step into history on the Lead Cove Trail, for what is a hike in the Smokies without a little human history? One theory states Lead Cove derived its name from ore that was extracted in the 1800s. If that was so, the operation was so small-scale as to be unseen today. Soon you pass an old homesite that lingers in the cool forest of the cove, bordered by Sugar Cove

 Historic Interest

61

Branch. Keep climbing and the hollow narrows, then you pass an unlikely chimney from a homesite at 0.5 mile.

At 0.7 mile, the hike turns away from Sugar Cove Branch. Slice through a ridgetop gap at 0.9 mile, then drift to Lead Cove Branch at 1.2 miles. Leave the water behind to arrive at Sandy Gap and the Bote Mountain Trail at mile 1.7. ▶2

R Stream

Turn right on the ridge to follow the former jeep trail of Bote Mountain. Ascend steadily through the fairly open pine-oak forest, slipping over to the east side of Coldwater Knob. Intermittent views of Defeat Ridge open to your left. At mile 2.9, pass through the Anthony Creek Trail junction. ▶3 Come to a jeep turnaround at mile 3.2. ▶4 The trail, dug out by generations of cows, horses, and people traveling a seemingly continuous rhododendron tunnel, becomes furrowed and narrow. Wind through a few switchbacks, passing trickling springs, to make a saddle on Spence Field at mile 4.6.

▲ Ridgeline

Turn left on the storied Appalachian Trail, ▶5 northbound, skirting Spence Field's eastern flank. The Spence Field backcountry shelter is right, a short distance away, on a spur trail. The trek to Rocky Top continues along the formerly large grassy meadow, now crowding in with haw, other trees,

TRAIL 7 Rocky Top via Lead Cove Elevation Profile

and rhododendron. Pass the Jenkins Ridge Trail, leaving right into North Carolina, at mile 4.9. ►6

Descend briefly only to begin the final 0.7 mile irregular climb to Rocky Top, 5,440 feet, and its rousing 360-degree view. ►7 Sandstone rock emerges from the soil and points toward the sky.

Once on top you'll understand why the view inspired a famed country song entitled "Rocky Top," which has become the fight song for the Volunteers of the University of Tennessee, a mere 30 miles away and visible on a clear day. To your west, the meadows of Spence Field and the western crest of the Smokies all the way to Shuckstack Mountain stand out in bold relief. The views into Tennessee and North Carolina stretch to the horizon. To your east the prominent peak with the imposing name "Thunderhead" competes with the sky. Embrace the view from this rock outcrop just as others have for generations. And maybe belt out a verse or two of "Rocky Top" before you leave.

 Great Views

 Autumn Colors

🚶	**MILESTONES**	
►1	0.0	Lead Cove Trailhead
►2	1.7	Right on Bote Mountain Trail
►3	2.9	Pass Anthony Creek Trail
►4	3.2	Old jeep turnaround
►5	4.6	Left on AT
►6	4.9	Pass Jenkins Ridge Trail
►7	5.8	Rocky Top

Finley Cane Loop

TRAIL 8

Whiteoak Sink

Schoolhouse Gap Trail

Meadow Branch

Turkeypen Ridge

Turkeypen Ridge Trail

Spence Branch

Schoolhouse Gap Trail

Laurel Creek

Turnback Branch

Bote Mountain Trail

West Prong Trail

P

start & finish

rock overhang

Pinkroot Branch

Laurel Creek Road

GREAT SMOKY MOUNTAINS NATIONAL PARK

Laurel Creek

Laurel Cove Creek

Bote Mountain Trail

Finley Cane Trail

Big Spring Cove

Crib Gap Trail

Lead Cove Trail

Hickory Tree Branch

Bote Mountain

Hickory Tree Gap

West Prong Little River

Devils Nest Creek

To Townsend, TN

Laurel Cove Creek

Sand Gap

Long Cove Creek

N

Sugar Cove Prong

0   0.2   0.4   0.6 miles

0   0.2   0.4   0.6 kilometers

Finley Cane Loop

Though you have to cross a road during this excursion, the trails on this hike are lightly used, offering a secluded undulating loop with no major elevation changes. Look for old homesites near quiet mountain streams. Gain obscured views while on piney ridges.

Best Time

This low-elevation hike is ideal for winter. You will also gain more views through leafless trees and spot old homesites better then. The many moist hollows are full of wildflowers in spring. Summer could be quite warm.

Finding the Trail

From Townsend, Tennessee, take TN 73 to enter the park. Turn right on Laurel Creek Road, toward Cades Cove, and follow it for 3.7 miles to the Schoolhouse Gap Trail parking area on your right.

Trail Description

This loop hike has no singular feature or destination. Rather it is simply a woodland walk through Smoky Mountain scenery that lives up to its national park status in a mostly secluded setting. The serenity adds value to the hike, as well as a few views, some pioneer homesites, and a variety of habitats ranging from piney ridges to rhododendron-choked hollows to cove hardwood forests. Plus no single climb or descent exceeding 400 feet.

TRAIL USE
Dayhiking, Horses

LENGTH
8.8 miles, 4–5½ hours

VERTICAL FEET
+900/-900

DIFFICULTY
– 1 2 **3** 4 5 +

TRAIL TYPE
Loop

FEATURES
Stream
Ridgeline
Autumn Colors
Wildflowers
Secluded
Historic Interest

FACILITIES
None

Walk around some large boulders at the trailhead ▶1 and pick up wide Schoolhouse Gap Trail. It briefly descends toward Laurel Creek, then turns up Spence Branch. Travel directly alongside the small clear stream as it flows over rock slabs in small stair-step cascades. The wide path is shaded by sycamores, witch hazel, and birches. Rhododendron finds its place as the trail heads up a cool, moist hollow. Bridge Spence Branch and continue at a gentle grade. The track suddenly steepens at 0.5 mile, after turning up a tributary of Spence Branch. Level off in a gap and high point at 0.8 mile. Cruise north to make Dorsey Gap and a trail junction at 1.1 miles. Here, the Turkeypen Ridge Trail leaves left, ▶2 while the Schoolhouse Gap Trail keeps straight.

⊳ Stream

▲ Ridgeline

Join narrow Turkeypen Ridge Trail. Wind your way along Turkeypen Ridge, exposing yourself to differing forest types, depending on the sun exposure in relation to the land. Occasionally cut through gaps in the ridgeline. Limited views open both north and south from the crest. South-facing slopes have various species of pine and mountain laurel, whereas the shaded ravines have black birch and rhododendron. The trail winds southwesterly. At 2.8 miles you are slipping in and out of drainages divided by rib ridges. At 3.4 miles, to the right of the

TRAIL 8 Finley Cane Loop Elevation Profile

trail, you will pass a prominent rock overhang with a spring flowing under it to Pinkroot Branch. ▶3

Continue winding over pine ridges and into moist ravines. At 4.2 miles, drift into Big Spring Cove. Watch for an overhang big enough to stand under right of the trail.

Step over Laurel Creek, then reach a four-way trail junction at 4.7 miles. Turn left here on the Crib Gap Trail, ▶4 passing through an old homes-ite. Reach a very unusual trail tunnel, which passes under Laurel Creek Road. Just ahead, reach another trail junction. Stay left, picking up the Finley Cane Trail, as a connector goes right to the Lead Cove Trail. Pass a dried up old pond in this formerly settled area. Watch for shortleaf pines invading the flats of Big Spring Cove.

 Historic Interest

Cross Laurel Cove Creek at 5.4 miles. The trail saddles up against Bote Mountain. From here the Finley Cane Trail features northern exposure type woodlands of tulip trees, sugar maple, and beech. Vines drape many trees. Cross many small wildflower-rich rills running perpendicular to the trail, flowing off Bote Mountain, between bisecting gaps dividing the streamsheds. Pass a horse-hitching post in a gap at 6.7 miles. ▶5 Just ahead is the trail's only stand of cane. Reach the route's high point just before meeting the Bote Mountain Trail at 7.3 miles. ▶6

Turn left on the wide path constructed by the first president of nearby Maryville College, Dr. Isaac Anderson. He built the road in the early 1800s to connect with settlements over on Hazel Creek in North Carolina, for Christian mission work. The road was built only to the state line, but then abandoned. The first 1.1 miles of the hike on Schoolhouse Gap Trail, was also part of what became known as Andersons Turnpike. Travel the dry ridge, enjoying southeasterly views of Defeat Ridge, across the gulf of West Prong Little River.

 Historic Interest

Take the West Prong Trail 0.6 mile to a backpack campsite for an overnight experience.

At 7.6 miles, the West Prong Trail leaves right 0.6 mile for West Prong backcountry campsite, #18. ▶7 Stay left with the Bote Mountain Trail, dipping into a rhododendron-filled hollow with a trickling stream in its center. Bridge the streamlet by culvert, then pop out on Laurel Creek Road at 8.8 miles. ▶8 The Schoolhouse Gap Trail parking area is to your left, about 50 yards down Laurel Creek Road.

🚶 MILESTONES

▶1	0.0	Schoolhouse Gap Trailhead
▶2	1.1	Left on Turkeypen Ridge Trail
▶3	3.4	Cross Pinkroot Branch
▶4	4.7	Left on Crib Gap Trail
▶5	6.7	Gap with horse-hitching post
▶6	7.3	Left on Bote Mountain Trail
▶7	7.6	West Prong Trail leaves right
▶8	8.8	Laurel Creek Road

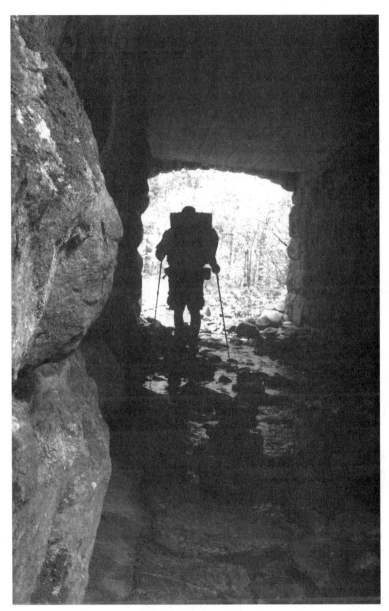

An unusual trail tunnel *passes under Laurel Creek Road.*

Tremont and Elkmont Area

Tremont and Elkmont Area

Tremont and Elkmont form the heart of the Tennessee Smokies. The hikes here are as varied as the elevation and include not only natural beauty but also historical destinations. Both dayhikes and overnight treks are included. Major highlights include fantastic vistas from the Appalachian Trail between Clingmans Dome and Silers Bald, the Smokies classic trek to The Chimneys, visits to waterfalls, and off-the-beaten-path getaways where nature reigns supreme.

Little River, easily one of the most scenic and largest watercourses in the Smokies, drains this diverse swath of Volunteer State mountain land. The headwaters of Little River flow north from Clingmans Dome and the state line crest, gathering volume from innumerable rills and branches. The biggest tributaries, Lynn Camp Prong and Middle Prong Little River, drain the Tremont area. The Tennessee and North Carolina state line forms the southern boundary. It is also where the Appalachian Trail runs, presenting some of the finest high country hiking in the Southeast. Newfound Gap Road splits the area to the east. The north side of the Little River Valley, cleaving the park from Wears Valley, encases Tremont and Elkmont.

The most extensive road and trailhead access in the Smokies and a huge biodiversity-creating elevation variation—from 6,642 feet at Clingmans Dome to 1,100 feet along the Little River—are upsides of the trail system here. Up high, spruce-fir forest adorns the crest from Newfound Gap westward to Silers Bald, and along the highest spur ridges. Northern hardwoods prevail below the Canadianesque evergreens, descending to reach the significant streams, which take on a more temperate vegetation as they crash deeper and lower. Here, notoriously dense forests rise, making the Smokies what they are. It is these temperate jungles that lead to the saying, "If it ain't movin', something's growin' on it." Pine and hardwoods such as oak thrive on south-facing, xeric sites.

Overleaf and opposite: Newfound Gap Road *as seen from The Chimney Tops (Trail 14)*

Auto access points start up top with seasonally open Clingmans Dome Road. Newfound Gap Road connects the high country to the Sugarlands Visitor Center, offering information, maps, books, and more. Little River Road heads west from the Sugarlands. First, it reaches Elkmont, a campground and major trailhead, before winding through the Little River gorge, connecting to Tremont. A separate, short motorway links Little River Road with Wears Valley. A dead-end road enters Tremont and provides more remote trail access. Two towns, Gatlinburg and Townsend, are conveniently situated nearby, but their proximity can be problematic during peak windshield-tourist seasons, such as summer holidays and fall weekends.

Historically speaking, this former Cherokee hunting ground gave way to settlers working their way deeper and deeper into the mountains, up the Little River valley, residing at simple farms and rude shacks. Settlement

Showy orchis *brightens the forest floor in spring along Little River (Trail 13).*

was never as thick as at places like Cades Cove, though one John Walker attempted to singlehandedly colonize Tremont with his multiple wives and scores of children. Some of the last residents of the Smokies, holdovers with lifetime leases, lived out their days here. Ol' Lem Ownby was the last man standing, along Jakes Creek above what is now Elkmont Campground. The Walker Sisters lived their days out in the Smokies. Their cabin is preserved and is a hiking destination described here. Ironically, the spinsters' home became a tourist stop so popular they wished for solitude late in life.

But large-scale logging ran Elkmont and Tremont settlers out before the park did. One W. B. Townsend, for whom the nearby town is named, began a railroad-based logging operation that nearly denuded Elkmont and Tremont. Eventually, Townsend sold his land to the park, but only with the agreement that he could continue logging for another 15 years. The amazing recuperative powers of nature are on display here, as verdant forests have risen to once again carpet the mountains. Later, Elkmont became a resort and summer home community, with some unoccupied houses still standing. Now, Elkmont is a major Smokies jumping-off point for tubers, anglers, campers, and equestrians. The Great Smoky Mountains Institute at Tremont adds an educational aspect to the area. Elkmont Campground is the major in-park overnight destination, though many area visitors lodge in Gatlinburg and Townsend. You might say Elkmont and Tremont are not only in the heart of the Tennessee side of the Smokies but are the pulse of the entire park.

Permits

Permits are *not* required for dayhiking. Backpackers, however, must get a backcountry permit to stay at one of the nine designated backcountry campsites and four trail shelters located here. Most require a simple self-registration; however, some campsites and all trail shelters require a reservation, which you can make by calling the backcountry permit office at (865) 436-1231. Pick up and fill out backcountry permits at the Great Smoky Mountains Institute in Tremont, Sugarlands Visitor Center near Gatlinburg, and the Elkmont campground office. If you're traveling in the high country, obtain your permit at Oconaluftee Visitor Center when coming from North Carolina or Sugarlands Visitor Center when coming from Tennessee.

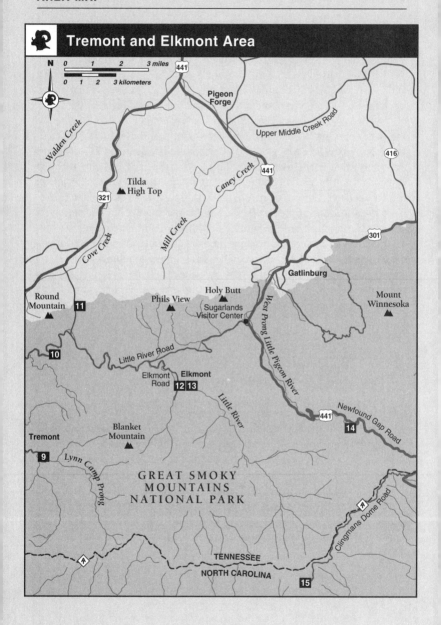

Tremont and Elkmont Area

N

0   1   2   3 miles

0   1   2   3 kilometers

441

Pigeon Forge

Upper Middle Creek Road

Walden Creek

416

Caney Creek

441

Tilda
High Top

321

301

Mill Creek

Cove Creek

Gatlinburg

Round Mountain

11

Phils View

Holy Butt

Sugarlands
Visitor Center

West Prong Little Pigeon River

Mount Winnesoka

10

Little River Road

Elkmont Road

Elkmont

12 13

Little River

441

Newfound Gap Road

14

Tremont

9

Lynn Camp Prong

Blanket Mountain

GREAT SMOKY
MOUNTAINS
NATIONAL PARK

Clingmans Dome Road

TENNESSEE

NORTH CAROLINA

15

Tremont and Elkmont Area

TRAIL	Difficulty	Length	Type	USES & ACCESS	TERRAIN	FLORA & FAUNA	OTHER
9	1	0.8	↗	👤 👥	Stream, Waterfall	Autumn Colors, Wildflowers	Swimming, Photo Opportunity, Historic Interest
10	2–3	6.8	↗	👤	Stream, Waterfall	Autumn Colors, Wildflowers	Swimming, Secluded
11	2	5.0	↗	👤	Stream, Mountain	Autumn Colors, Wildflowers	Great Views, Historic Interest
12	2–3	5.6	↻	👤	Stream, Summit, Waterfall	Autumn Colors, Wildflowers	Swimming, Historic Interest
13	3	7.8	↗	👤 🏇	Stream, Waterfall	Autumn Colors, Wildflowers	Swimming, Historic Interest
14	3	4.0	↗	👤	Stream, Mountain	Autumn Colors, Wildflowers, Old-growth	Great Views, Swimming, Steep, Photo Opportunity
15	3	9.6	↗	👤 🏇	Mountain	Autumn Colors, Wildflowers, Spruce-fir	Great Views, Photo Opportunity

USES & ACCESS	TYPE	TERRAIN	FLORA & FAUNA	FEATURES
👤 Dayhiking	↻ Loop	⛰ Mountain	🍁 Autumn Colors	💪 Great Views
🏇 Backpacking	↗ Out & Back	△ Summit	❋ Wildflowers	📷 Photo Opportunity
🐴 Horses	↘ Point-to-Point	▲ Ridgeline	🦌 Wildlife	⚠ Backcountry Camping
👥 Child Friendly	DIFFICULTY - 1 2 3 4 5 + less more	⫿ Stream	🌲 Spruce-fir	⚓ Swimming
		⫿⫿ Waterfall	🌳 Old-growth	🎯 Secluded
		≈ Lake		⬇ Steep
				🏠 Historic Interest
				🔨 Geologic Interest

Maps

For the Tremont and Elkmont area, here are the USGS 7.5-minute (1:24,000-scale) topographic quadrangles that you will need, listed in the order that you will need them as you hike along your route.

  Trail 9: Thunderhead Mountain
  Trail 10: Wear Cove
  Trail 11: Wear Cove
  Trail 12: Gatlinburg
  Trail 13: Gatlinburg, Silers Bald
  Trail 14: Mount Le Conte, Clingmans Dome
  Trail 15: Clingmans Dome, Silers Bald

Tremont and Elkmont Area

Cucumber Gap Loop 97

TRAIL 12

Dayhiking
5.6 miles, Loop
Difficulty: 1 **2** 3 4 5

Leave Elkmont and cruise up the ultra-attractive Little River valley, where the watercourse tumbles over huge boulders, forming large, clear pools that invite a dip in the cool mountain stream. Pass a tributary waterfall. Leave the Little River on an old railroad grade that gently climbs to a gap and then descends to Jakes Creek Valley, returning to Elkmont.

Little River Hike 103

TRAIL 13

Dayhiking, Backpacking
7.8 miles, Out & Back
Difficulty: 1 2 **3** 4 5

This hike wanders up the Little River valley, featuring everywhere-you-look national park beauty. The trek ends at an iron bridge overlooking the Little River, but your walk can be shortened or extended depending on company and circumstances.

The Chimney Tops 107

TRAIL 14

Dayhiking
4.0 miles, Out & Back
Difficulty: 1 2 **3** 4 5

This busy and steep hike is nothing less than spectacular. Cross chilly mountain streams on a series of footbridges to ascend sharply amid some old trees. Emerge at the Smokies single most recognizable rock formation: the twin spires of the Chimney Tops, which provide a dramatic view of the surrounding landscape.

Silers Bald via Clingmans Dome 111

TRAIL 15

Dayhiking, Backpacking
9.6 miles, Out & Back
Difficulty: 1 2 **3** 4 5

Begin at the park's highest trailhead, near Clingmans Dome, and follow the Appalachian Trail along a knife-edge ridge. Roller-coaster along the spine of the Smokies, presenting stellar views. Reach the fast disappearing field of Silers Bald, enjoying multiple vistas.

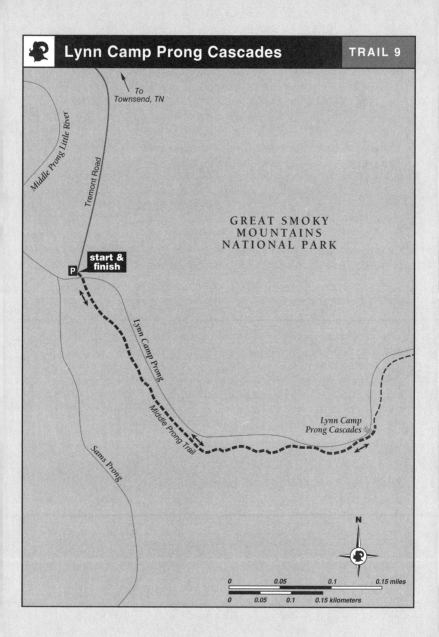

Lynn Camp Prong Cascades   TRAIL 9

To
Townsend, TN

Middle Prong Little River

Tremont Road

start &
finish
P

GREAT SMOKY
MOUNTAINS
NATIONAL PARK

Lynn Camp Prong

Middle Prong Trail

Sams Prong

Lynn Camp
Prong Cascades

N

0   0.05   0.1   0.15 miles

0   0.05   0.1   0.15 kilometers

Lynn Camp Prong Cascades

This easy family stroll follows a quintessential mountain stream. Take a wide and easy track along scenic Lynn Camp Prong. Enjoy a forest montage of a valley that was once the site of a logging community. Reach an observation bench with a straight-on view of the cataract. The falls can be accessed from here or a little farther on up the trail.

Best Time

This short hike is good for all seasons. Spring wildflowers will be rife in the valley, and the stream will be at its boldest. In summer, the stream will avail an ideal cooling place. In winter you will best see evidence of the former logging community.

Finding the Trail

From Townsend, Tennessee, take TN 73 to enter the park at the Townsend Wye. Turn right on Laurel Creek Road and follow it for 0.2 mile then turn left into Tremont. Follow Tremont Road past the Tremont Environmental Education Center, where it turns to gravel, to dead end after a total of 5.1 miles. The Middle Prong Trail starts at the upper end of the parking area.

Trail Description

When visiting the Smokies, we see the park in its current state. Sometimes it is hard to imagine what it once was. Along this hike you could envision the time when the Middle Prong Little River was

TRAIL USE
Dayhiking,
    Child Friendly

LENGTH
0.8 mile, 1 hour

VERTICAL FEET
+150/-150

DIFFICULTY
– **1** 2 3 4 5 +

TRAIL TYPE
Out & Back

FEATURES
Stream
Waterfall
Autumn Colors
Wildflowers
Swimming
Historic
Photo Opportunity

FACILITIES
None

81

the forest primeval—a place where uncut giants stretched for the mountaintops, where nature's hand placed a dizzying array of trees and lesser flora just so, where bear, elk, bison, and red wolves vied for supremacy. Or you could imagine a place where John Walker and his numerous wives—and numerous offspring—populated this valley that came to be known as Tremont. Picture rudimentary log cabins in sunlit clearings, where a stone chimney pushed smoke above a plot of overturned soil, waiting for spring to begin. Or you could conceive what took place just before this locale became part of the Great Smoky Mountains National Park—one of the first railroad-driven, massive-scale, no-holds-barred logging operations in the South, undertaken from the late 1920s to the late 30s, an operation so complete and efficient for the time it shocked and stunned even those involved.

Today, on this trek you will see nature's beauty standing the test of time, and the amazing recuperative powers of these Tennessee woods. You will also see remnants of the Little River Lumber Company and its push up the valley in a quest for some of the largest uncut forests in the country.

The access road to the trailhead and the trail itself follow the old logging rail originally graded by

TRAIL 9 Lynn Camp Prong Cascades Elevation Profile

the lumber company. Northern timber interests had perfected railroad-based, steam-engine-powered logging and set their sights on the uncut verdant forests of the Smokies. And they came in using not only the latest machinery but also a new efficiency that moved men and their families wherever the cutting was to be done. The trailhead was once the community of Tremont.

After parking, walk around and picture a simple community building functioning as the school, the church, and movie theater—the center of group events. The employees lived in portable shacks that were moved by the railroad and offloaded by steam shovels. These steam-powered machines were used primarily to load cut logs onto the railcars. There was a railroad siding area, where cars were taken on and off the train. The movable homes were located in the flat. A water-powered generator provided electricity to the community.

Now, begin your walk, ►1 crossing the arched steel bridge over Lynn Camp Prong, just above its confluence with Sams Prong. Together they form the Middle Prong Little River. Just across the bridge was another part of the community. Here stood the company store, where employees paid their bills in scrip, a unit of value issued by the company for employees to buy supplies. The post office was in the store as well. A rudimentary doctor's office stood near Lynn Camp Prong.

 Historic Interest

Rail lines went up Sams Prong and Lynn Camp Prong. Your hike goes left here, up Lynn Camp Prong. The grade is steep for a train. Only gear-driven locomotives were used to push the cars up empty and slowly work them back down to the sawmill in Townsend.

Imagine what a noisy, rumbling place this would've been. But, even amidst the logging chaos, the Smokies splendor was undeniable. In the flat across the river, the Tremont Hotel was established.

Originally for employees of the logging outfit, it later offered tourists lodging and hot meals. The hotel was dismantled with the coming of the park and is now just a picture and a memory.

Wildflowers

Leave the logging world behind, continuing on up the trail. The forest is once again magnificent and should continue to flourish. The moist valley is an ideal wildflower habitat. The wide track allows hikers to trek side-by-side in conversation while appreciating the scenery. At 0.4 mile, you come to a contemplation bench facing Lynn Camp Prong Cascades. ▶2

Waterfall

Lynn Camp Prong *crashes in a white froth over a rock face.*

The cataract leaves an upstream pool, then fills a rock-lined channel, building up energy. It then is unleashed, tumbling down a stone face in white froth. A jumble of rocks, left over from blasting the rail line, lie between you and the falls, but hikers make it to the base of the falls for an up-close view of Lynn Camp Prong. Others continue along the trail, and reach the upper end of the fall and the stone face over which it tumbles. This upper vantage complements the view from the bench.

Photo Opportunity

You will also see more cascades upstream of the main fall. Together they add up to more than 80 feet tall! When adding together the ceaseless waterfall, flowing through all the changes of Tremont, the rising forests making a national park level comeback, and the pioneer lives led in this neck of the woods, followed by the loggers and their portable world, the locale really is a place for contemplation.

🚶	**MILESTONES**		
▶1	0.0	Middle Prong Trailhead
▶2	0.4	Lynn Camp Prong Cascades

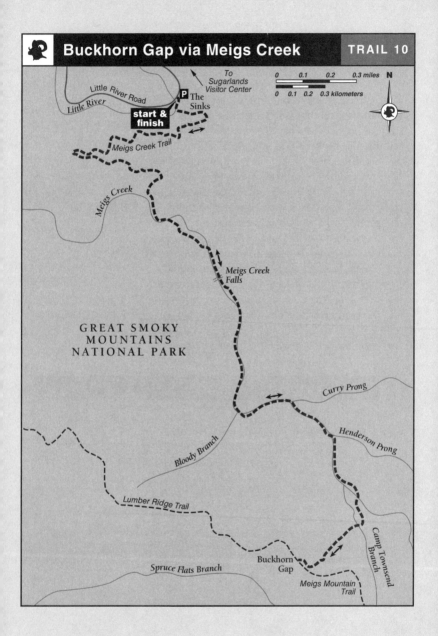

To
Sugarlands
Visitor Center

Little River Road

Little River

P

start &
finish

The
Sinks

Meigs Creek Trail

0   0.1   0.2   0.3 miles

0   0.1   0.2   0.3 kilometers

N

Meigs Creek

Meigs Creek
Falls

GREAT SMOKY
MOUNTAINS
NATIONAL PARK

Curry Prong

Henderson Prong

Bloody Branch

Lumber Ridge Trail

Camp Townsend Branch

Spruce Flats Branch

Buckhorn
Gap

Meigs Mountain
Trail

Buckhorn Gap via Meigs Creek

From the popular waterfall and swimming area of the Sinks on the Little River, take the quiet Meigs Creek Trail over a ridge with views. Join Meigs Creek to view a waterfall. Numerous creek crossings of Meigs Creek and its tributaries lead through a gorgeous and secluded valley to wooded Buckhorn Gap.

TRAIL USE
Dayhiking

LENGTH
6.8 miles, 3½–4½ hours

VERTICAL FEET
+980/-980

DIFFICULTY
– 1 **2** 3 4 5 +

TRAIL TYPE
Out & Back

FEATURES
Stream
Waterfall
Autumn Colors
Wildflowers
Swimming
Secluded

FACILITIES
None

Best Time

You will have to make nearly 20 rock-hop crossings of Meigs Creek and its tributaries on this trek. Late summer and fall offer the lowest water and easiest crossings. However, the waterfall of the Sinks and Meigs Creek Falls is less spectacular then. Consider coming during early summer when you can wet your feet without penalty and enjoy bolder cascades. During spring, the Meigs Creek valley can be a wildflower wonderland.

Finding the Trail

From Sugarlands Visitor Center, drive 12 miles east on the Little River Road to the Sinks parking area on your left. The Meigs Creek Trail starts at the rear of the parking area.

Trail Description

After leaving the crowds at the Sinks behind, you'll probably have this intimate slice of the Smokies to yourself. The smaller subtle features of a Southern Appalachian mountain valley stand out on this trail. Meigs Creek will surely catch your eye, as you cross it nearly 20 times. Not to worry though, as most crossings are not difficult in times of normal water flow.

Leave the revamped Sinks parking area, ▶1 leading to a wide path and a viewing platform overlooking the falls feeding the Sinks, a large pool popular with swimmers. The signed Meigs Creek Trail begins on stone steps beyond the platform. Pass a natural rock promontory overlooking the Sinks. Once on the Meigs Creek Trail drop into a boggy area, unusual for the Smokies. Black birch, white pine, and tulip trees grow tall and lush. A slender path rises past rock outcrops as it winds into small tributaries. Ascend onto a dry piney ridge, leveling off at 0.9 mile ▶2 amid sassafras, sourwood, and oaks, a forest change from the Little River valley. In winter views of Meigs Creek open to the south. Wind back down to finally encounter the trail's namesake, Meigs Creek, at 1.4 miles. ▶3

Here begin the crossings, as the creek and trail merge amid a dark green forest interspersed with crashing cascades that flow beneath tunnels of rhododendron above which rise black birch. Rock-hop your way across the stream. At 1.7 miles, a particularly comely cascades, Meigs Creek Falls, announces its presence on your right. It spills over a sheer stone face 15 feet into a pool. Beyond the falls,

▌ Waterfall

M Great Views

▶ Stream

▌ Waterfall

TRAIL 10 Buckhorn Gap via Meigs Creek Elevation Profile

continue fording. While crossing, notice the clarity of the stream.

At 2.0 miles, on trail left, look for the first of two huge beech trees. ►4 Buckeyes grow tall in this valley, which also once harbored massive hemlocks. Selective loggers left these hemlock trees behind. They were not considered commercially valuable in the early 20th century and were left to become the giants of the forest they are today, ultimately to fall prey to the hemlock wooly adelgid. As you continue a moderate uptick, Meigs Creek and the side creeks that feed it shrink, but still display an array of scenic shoals, slides, and pools amid mossy logs, gray boulders, and overhanging rhododendron.

Rock-hop tributaries in the upper valley. The final climb at 3.3 miles signals your impending arrival at Buckhorn Gap. ►5 Once at the gap, you intersect the Meigs Mountain Trail, which goes left to Elkmont, and the Lumber Ridge Trail, which goes to Tremont. Take a seat at the gap and listen to the sounds of the Smokies before returning to the busy Sinks.

The people who settled these isolated coves revered their moving water and couldn't cotton to drinking "still" well water after they left their highland homes.

⋏	**MILESTONES**	
►1	0.0	The Sinks parking area
►2	0.9	Ridgetop with views
►3	1.4	First crossing of Meigs Creek
►4	2.0	Huge beech trees
►5	3.4	Buckhorn Gap

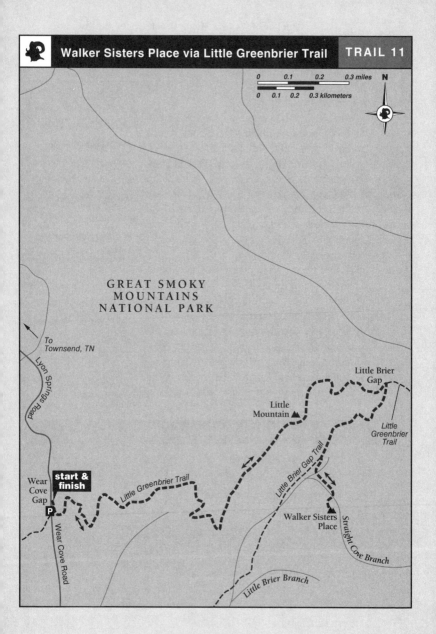

Walker Sisters Place via Little Greenbrier Trail   TRAIL 11

0   0.1   0.2   0.3 miles   N

0   0.1   0.2   0.3 kilometers

GREAT SMOKY
MOUNTAINS
NATIONAL PARK

To
Townsend, TN

Lyon Springs Road

Little Brier
Gap

Little
Mountain ▲

Little
Greenbrier
Trail

start &
finish

Wear
Cove
Gap

P

Little Greenbrier Trail

Little Brier Gap Trail

Walker Sisters
Place

Straight Cove Branch

Wear Cove Road

Little Brier Branch

Walker Sisters Place via Little Greenbrier Trail

Soak up some views and then visit one of the last working pioneer homesteads in the Smokies. Trace the Little Greenbrier Trail as it straddles the national park boundary. Vistas are numerous from a pine-cloaked mountainside before reaching a gap. Descend a hollow and reach the Walker Sisters Place, occupied by spinster siblings until 1964.

TRAIL USE
Dayhiking
LENGTH
5.0 miles, 3 hours
VERTICAL FEET
+400/-300
DIFFICULTY
− 1 **2** 3 4 5 +
TRAIL TYPE
Out & Back

FEATURES
Ridgeline
Stream
Autumn Colors
Wildflowers
Great Views
Historic

FACILITIES
None

Best Time

Since it is a relatively low-elevation hike, winter is favorable. Spring is also a good choice, when Little Brier Branch comes alive with wildflowers. Fall brings clear skies and dry trails.

Finding the Trail

From the park entrance at Townsend, head straight to the Townsend Wye, a split in the road. Turn left here, onto Little River Road, and follow it for 7.8 miles to Metcalf Bottoms Picnic Area. Turn left into Metcalf Bottoms Picnic Area, crossing the Little River on a bridge. Keep on the road for 1.3 miles to the park border, where the Little Greenbrier Trail starts on the right. There is parking here for only one car directly by the trail; another parking area is just over the hill from the trailhead.

Trail Description

This hike travels a ridgeline that seemingly divides time periods in East Tennessee. On one side there is the preserved Great Smoky Mountains National

Park, where the Walker Sisters Cabin, your destination, exemplifies a simpler time, when the Smokies were truly the back of beyond, where homesteaders would spend a lifetime and never get more than 100 miles from home. On the other side of the ridge modern "homesteaders" stake vacation homes in Wears Valley to be near the beauty that is the national park, changing Wears Valley from a land of the forgotten to an urban outpost. Your mind may contemplate such things while wandering the ridge known as Little Mountain, the northern border of the Smokies.

Begin this hike at Wear Cove Gap on the Little Greenbrier Trail. ▶1 Climb through archetypal pine, oak, and mountain laurel forest on a narrow pathway. Blueberries are abundant in sunnier locales. This path skirts the park border in several places; you will see boundary signs here and there. Also, observe elaborate stonework by trail makers that keeps the path from sliding down the mountainside. Views open north beyond the park, especially at a gap at 0.5 mile. ▶2

H Great Views

▲ Ridgeline

Hike more up than down then curve around the south side of Little Mountain at 1.0 mile. Listen for flowing water in the lowlands below. Enjoy good looks into the park's heart. Numerous dead pine snags are the result of natural relationships

TRAIL 11 Walker Sisters Place via Little Greenbrier Trail Elevation Profile

between pines and the native pine beetle. The snags are now falling and younger trees are taking their place. The walking is easy, allowing you to enjoy more views into Wear Cove and Cove Mountain to the east. Descend the ridge of Little Mountain to reach Little Brier Gap and a trail junction at mile 1.9. ▶3 Turn right here, joining the Little Brier Gap Trail, descending into the moist cove of Little Brier Branch. Tulip trees join the forest.

Great Views

Autumn Colors

Wildflowers

Walker Sisters Place *is one of the better preserved homesteads in the park.*

Stream

Historic Interest

The V-shaped hollow widens. Little Brier Branch gains flow from tributaries. Reach a signed trail junction at 2.3 miles. ►4 The Little Brier Gap Trail continues as a gravel road while a spur track leads left to the Walker Sisters Place. Turn left along tiny Straight Cove Branch. The preponderance of tulip trees and shortleaf pines indicate former fields. Imagine these trailside flats growing corn and other vegetables, perhaps as pasture, back when this was an active homestead. Come to an open area at 2.5 miles and reach the Walker Sisters Place in a grassy clearing. ►5 This cove was occupied for 150 years, with the Walker Sisters remaining after the national park was established, thanks to a lifetime lease agreement. After they passed away, the park preserved their homestead. Now, the springhouse, main home, and small barn remain.

Notice the notched-log construction of the buildings and the nonnative ornamental bushes. Walk inside. The low roof required less construction material and also made the home easier to heat. The white stuff on the walls is old pieces of newspaper that the sisters used to brighten and insulate the cabin. A ladder leads to the sleeping loft. The large fireplace warmed the home, and heat rising up the rock "chimbley" kept loft sleepers a little toastier. The springhouse kept critters from fouling the water and also helped milk and butter stay cool in the summertime. The barn is a smaller version of the cantilever-type popular in East Tennessee a century and more ago. Note the farm implements on the wall.

Walk the perimeter of the yard, and you will see other relics, including old car tires, that the Walker Sisters likely regarded as junk. Remember to leave all artifacts so others can enjoy and discover them. If you are further interested in the area's history, continue down the Little Brier Gap Trail for 1.1 more miles to the Little Greenbrier Schoolhouse before returning to Wear Cove Gap.

MILESTONES

▶1	0.0	Little Greenbrier Trailhead
▶2	0.5	Gap with views
▶3	1.9	Right on Little Brier Gap Trail
▶4	2.3	Left on spur to Walker Sisters Place
▶5	2.5	Walker Sisters Place

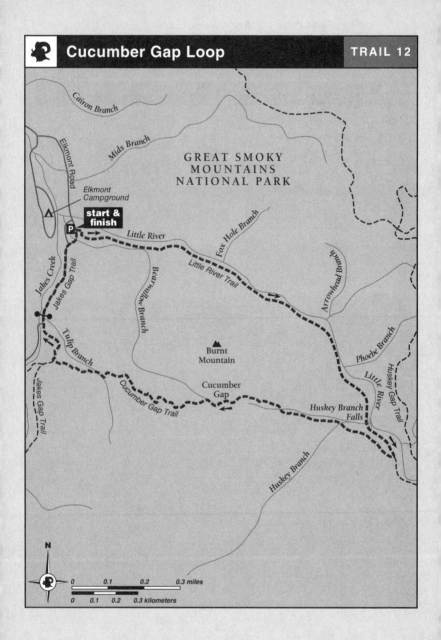

Cucumber Gap Loop

TRAIL 12

Cairon Branch

Elkmont Road

Mids Branch

GREAT SMOKY
MOUNTAINS
NATIONAL PARK

Elkmont
Campground

start & finish

P

Little River

Fox Hole Branch

Arrowhead Branch

Jakes Creek

Jakes Gap Trail

Little River Trail

Bearwallow Branch

Burnt
Mountain

Phoebe Branch

Tulip Branch

Little River

Huskey Gap Trail

Jakes Gap Trail

Cucumber Gap Trail

Cucumber
Gap

Huskey Branch
Falls

Huskey Branch

N

| 0 | 0.1 | 0.2 | 0.3 miles |
| 0 | 0.1 | 0.2 | 0.3 kilometers |

Cucumber Gap Loop

Leave Elkmont and cruise up the ultra-attractive Little River valley, where the watercourse tumbles over huge boulders, forming large, clear pools that invite a dip in the cool mountain stream. Pass a tributary waterfall. Leave the Little River on an old railroad grade that gently climbs to a gap and then descends to Jakes Creek Valley, returning to Elkmont.

TRAIL USE
Dayhiking
LENGTH
5.6 miles, 3 hours
VERTICAL FEET
+880/-880
DIFFICULTY
– 1 **2 3** 4 5 +
TRAIL TYPE
Loop

Best Time

This is a great hike year-round. In spring wildflowers abound along the Little River and Huskey Branch. Swimmers and sunbathers can enjoy the big waters of the Little River. Fall colors are vibrant along the streams and near Cucumber Gap. Solitude seekers will enjoy winter.

FEATURES
Waterfall
Stream
Ridgeline
Autumn Colors
Wildflowers
Swimming
Historic

Finding the Trail

From Sugarlands Visitor Center near Gatlinburg, turn right onto Little River Road and follow it 4.9 miles then turn left into Elkmont. Follow the paved road 1.3 miles to Elkmont Campground. Turn left just before the campground check-in station, and follow this road a short distance to cross the Little River. The Little River Trail starts on the left shortly after the bridge.

FACILITIES
Campground
Picnic tables
Restrooms
Water

Trail Description

The Little River Trail's beginning was once part of Little River Road until a mid-1990s flood washed

Historic Interest

Stream

Wildflowers

out this upper section. The park service decided to move the trailhead ▶1 back rather than repair the road. Pass through the former Elkmont summer home community, formerly known as the Appalachian Club, on a crumbling asphalt path. Vestiges of the stone entry gates and summer cottages survive. After a quarter mile you leave the old summer cottage community on a wide gravel track shaded by tulip trees, sycamore, black birch, yellow birch over scads of doghobble, and rhododendron mixed with mossy boulders. The sparkling Little River to the left constantly tries to lure you to its banks with attractive shoals, crystalline pools, small islands, and big rocks ideal for sunning or feeling the cool breeze flow down the valley. A dip may be in order during the dog days of summer. At 0.4 mile, Bearwallow Branch comes in on your right.

At 1.0 mile, the path narrows after you pass the old parking area. A bluff pinches the trail to the river in places. In other spots the Little River is only audible, not visible. The Little River drains the highest point in the Smokies, Clingmans Dome, then gathers tributaries, flowing north and west through the park before emerging near the community of Townsend. The watercourse continues northwest to meet the Tennessee River near Maryville. In the park, intrepid

TRAIL 12 Cucumber Gap Loop Elevation Profile

kayakers tackle its white froth during higher flows. Foolish tubers get injured every summer floating it. You can enjoy more casual canoeing and kayaking nearly year-round along its lower reaches.

Burnt Mountain rises to your right; this hike leads completely around that wooded peak. At 2.0 miles, Huskey Branch flows beneath a bridge into the Little River and a large pool below. Here, Huskey Branch tumbles as a tiered cascade above and below the trail as it slices through jagged rock. ▶2 Look into the pool below Huskey Branch for swimming trout. Brook trout, technically a char, are the only native trout in the Smokies. However, brown trout and rainbow trout have been introduced into the park and thrive in its waters. In the lower Little River you are most likely to see brown and rainbow trout.

Keep walking for a bit, coming to an intersection with the Cucumber Gap Trail at 2.4 miles. ▶3 Turn right onto the Cucumber Gap Trail. This path may have more vines among the trees than any other trail in the park. Ascend an old railroad grade, rockhopping Huskey Branch at mile 2.8. ▶4 Muscadine vines are prominent elements of the trailside forest. The small native grapes ripen in early fall and are favored by all sorts of wildlife in the Smokies. The thick-skinned fruit grows throughout the Southeast; early settlers used it to make wine. Today winemakers cultivate the varietal. The antioxidant-laden fruit is also touted as a modern-day health food.

The path keeps rising along a small feeder stream of Huskey Branch, crossing the tributary at 3.2 miles. Occasional views open through the trees to the right. The path passes just above Cucumber Gap at 3.5 miles, you are just below 3,000 feet. ▶5 The gap was named for the cucumber tree, which is part of the magnolia family. Its green fruit resembles a mini-cucumber and can be seen trailside in September. The tree appears throughout the

Waterfall

Stream

Autumn Colors

mid-Appalachians, with West Virginia in the heart of its range. Outlier populations stretch to Louisiana and Missouri.

Historic Interest

The flat in Cucumber Gap was once home to a Smoky Mountain pioneer family. Look for leveled locations and piled stones in the woods, perhaps reminiscent of those people. Pass some fairly large beech trees and arrow-straight regal tulip trees before descending to cross Tulip Branch at 4.4 miles.

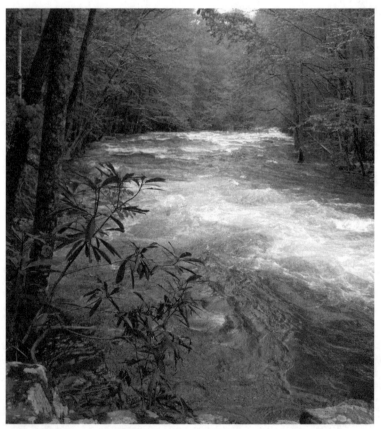

Little River *charges downstream following heavy spring rains.*

Meet the wide Jakes Creek Trail at 4.6 miles. ▶6 Turn right here and descend to a pole gate at 5.0 miles. Enter the former summer home community, passing the Jakes Creek Trailhead parking area. ▶7 Keep downhill on an asphalt path to the Jakes Creek Trailhead at mile 5.5. ▶8 Turn right here, follow the paved road, and soon reach the Little River Trailhead, completing your loop at 5.6 miles. ▶9

🚶	MILESTONES	
▶1	0.0	Little River Trailhead
▶2	2.0	Huskey Branch waterfall
▶3	2.4	Right on Cucumber Gap Trail
▶4	2.8	Cross Huskey Branch
▶5	3.5	Cucumber Gap
▶6	4.6	Right on Jakes Creek Trail
▶7	5.0	Jakes Creek Trailhead
▶8	5.5	Right at road split
▶9	5.6	Little River Trailhead

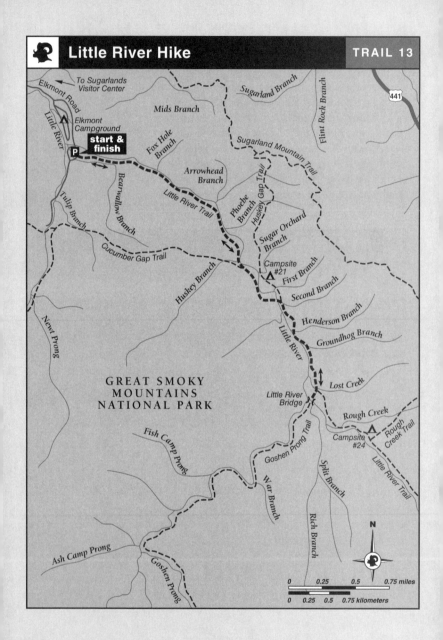

Little River Hike

441

To Sugarlands Visitor Center

Elkmont Road

Little River

Elkmont Campground

start & finish

P

Sugarland Branch

Flint Rock Branch

Mids Branch

Fox Hole Branch

Sugarland Mountain Trail

Arrowhead Branch

Little River Trail

Phoebe Branch

Huskey Gap Trail

Sugar Orchard Branch

Tulip Branch

Bearwallow Branch

Cucumber Gap Trail

Huskey Branch

Campsite #21

First Branch

Second Branch

Henderson Branch

New Prong

Little River

Groundhog Branch

GREAT SMOKY MOUNTAINS NATIONAL PARK

Lost Creek

Little River Bridge

Rough Creek

Campsite #24

Rough Creek Trail

Fish Camp Prong

Goshen Prong Trail

War Branch

Split Branch

Little River Trail

Rich Branch

Ash Camp Prong

Goshen Prong

N

| 0 | 0.25 | 0.5 | 0.75 miles |
| 0 | 0.25 | 0.5 | 0.75 kilometers |

Little River Hike

This hike wanders up the Little River valley, featuring everywhere-you-look national park beauty. The trek ends at an iron bridge overlooking the Little River, but your walk can be shortened or extended depending on company and circumstances.

Best Time

This hike is good year-round. In winter bold Little River may be bordered by ice and snow. Wildflowers run rampant in the valley in spring. Summer can be good for fishing, swimming, and cooling off. The varied deciduous woodland are vibrant with color in fall.

Finding the Trail

From Sugarlands Visitor Center near Gatlinburg, turn right onto Little River Road and follow it 4.9 miles then turn left into Elkmont. Follow the paved road 1.3 miles to Elkmont Campground. Turn left just before the campground check-in station, and follow this road a short distance to cross Little River. Little River Trail starts on the left shortly after the bridge.

Trail Description

I ran into a woman on this trail and asked her why she was on it. She pointed her finger and simply said, "By the river." This hike gently follows the Little River deep into the heart of the Smokies, in the shadow of Clingmans Dome. Your destination is a bridge spanning the Little River. Along the way, you see the stream at its finest, deep in the bosom of the park.

TRAIL USE
Dayhiking, Backpacking

LENGTH
7.8 miles, 3–5 hours

VERTICAL FEET
+560/-560

DIFFICULTY
– 1 2 **3** 4 5 +

TRAIL TYPE
Out & Back

FEATURES
Stream
Waterfall
Autumn Colors
Wildflowers
Swimming
Historic Interest

FACILITIES
Camping
Water

The cascading watercourse presents an ever-changing water show. The Little River crashes amid water-worn boulders, only to gather in large pools to fall again in a white, frothy mix of water and air.

Leave the parking area, ▶1 passing through the old cottage community known as the Appalachian Club. It was mostly peopled from nearby Knoxville, Tennessee, from where in early days they would take a train to this parcel of the Smokies. Later, the Little River Lumber Company abruptly pulled up its tracks, and members of the Appalachian Club banded together and had a road built over the railroad grade extending from Townsend to Elkmont.

After a quarter mile, leave the community and continue up the continuously stunning Little River. Pass Bearwallow Branch at 0.4 mile. The path reaches a former trailhead at 1.0 mile, then narrows. At mile 2.0, Huskey Branch enters the Little River in a waterfall above the trail. ▶2 The creek then runs under the trail and spills into the Little River. A deep pool trout-filled pool swirls below.

You will intersect the Cucumber Gap Trail at 2.4 miles. ▶3 Keep straight on the Little River Trail, crossing it on a wide wooden bridge just before meeting the Huskey Gap Trail at mile 2.8. ▶4 Stay on the east bank of the Little River, crossing several small feeder streams originating from Sugarland

Historic Interest

Stream

Waterfall

Autumn Colors

TRAIL 13 Little River Hike Elevation Profile

Backpacking

OPTIONS

If you stay straight on the Little River Trail, you can wander into the Rough Creek backcountry campsite, #24, at mile 4.6. The Little River Trail becomes somewhat rougher and rockier as it passes the Rough Creek trail junction just beyond the Rough Creek campsite. Look for the even spacing of old railroad ties, left over from the logging days. Arrive at the Three Forks back-country campsite, #30, elevation 3,400, at 6.4 miles. It was once a logging camp. The Three Forks are the Little River, Grouse Creek, and Spud Town Branch. The Grouse Creek Valley must've been particularly rough on the loggers or settlers who roamed this back of beyond. Listen to these tributary names of Grouse Creek: Rattler Branch, Devil Branch, and Snake Tongue Branch!

Mountain: Second Branch, Henderson Branch, and Groundhog Branch. Great views of the main river open. Come to a wide, wooded flat and trail junction at 3.8 miles. ▶5

Turn right here on the Goshen Prong Trail. Travel a straight, old railroad grade to soon reach an iron bridge over the Little River. ▶6 Hikers can see the confluence of Fish Camp Prong and Little River below the iron bridge. A large pool gathers here, great for swimming. Upstream you can see the Little River braiding around an island. This place's subtle yet sublime beauty make it one of my favorite places in the Great Smoky Mountains.

Little River used to be one of the park's harder fords.

🏊● Swimming

🚶	MILESTONES	
▶1	0.0	Little River Trailhead
▶2	2.0	Huskey Branch waterfall
▶3	2.4	Pass Cucumber Gap Trail
▶4	2.8	Huskey Gap Trail leaves left
▶5	3.8	Right on Goshen Prong Trail
▶6	3.9	Bridge over Little River

The Chimney Tops

TRAIL 14

N

0   0.1   0.2   0.3 miles
0   0.1   0.2   0.3 kilometers

West Prong Little Pigeon River

To Sugarlands Visitor Center

441

Newfound Gap Road

start & finish

P

Road Prong Trail

GREAT SMOKY MOUNTAINS NATIONAL PARK

Chimney Tops

rock scramble

Road Prong

Chimney Tops Trail

Road Prong Trail

The Chimney Tops

This busy and steep hike is nothing less than spectacular. Cross chilly mountain streams on a series of footbridges to ascend sharply amid some old trees. Emerge at the Smokies single most recognizable rock formation: the twin spires of the Chimney Tops, which provide a dramatic view of the surrounding landscape.

Best Time

This hike is good year-round but is crowded during the warm weather season. Try to go during off-times. In spring, fall, and winter you enjoy the best views. Avoid this hike during summer altogether unless you can hike at dawn or dusk.

Finding the Trail

From Sugarlands Visitor Center, take Newfound Gap Road 6.7 miles. The Chimney Tops parking area is on your right, just after a tunnel.

Trail Description

If you don't mind some company on the trail, this short but steep hike is nothing less than spectacular. Leave Newfound Gap Road and its cars behind on a series of footbridges over crystalline streams. Ascend sharply amid some old trees to come out on top of the Smokies most recognizable rock formation: the twin spires of the Chimney Tops, which provide a dramatic view of the surrounding landscape.

TRAIL USE
Dayhiking

LENGTH
4.0 miles, 2–3 hours

VERTICAL FEET
+1,200/-1,200

DIFFICULTY
– 1 2 **3** 4 5 +

TRAIL TYPE
Out & Back

FACILITIES
Stream
Ridgeline
Autumn Colors
Wildflowers
Swimming
Great Views
Steep
Old-growth
Geologic Interest
Photo Opportunity

FACILITIES
None

This steep trail starts by going down. Leave the parking area ▶1 on the Chimney Tops Trail and follow the path down to Walker Camp Prong, where a footbridge awaits your crossing. The white cataract with a big pool attracts swimmers on a hot day. Continue on, entering Beech Flats Cove. Northern hardwoods of beech, silverbell, and yellow birch complement some preserved hemlocks to cross Road Prong on two footbridges in short succession. Just after the fourth footbridge, you'll come to the Road Prong Trail junction, at 0.9 mile. ▶2 It leaves left for the state line ridge, and once was an historic crossing between Tennessee and North Carolina.

Turn right, staying on the Chimney Tops Trail, which steepens considerably. Due to the heavy traffic, the trail is rutted and has toe-grabbing roots along the way. Watch your step, but don't forget to look up every now and then to admire the old-growth trees, buckeye among them, which accompany your ascent. Hikers will be standing beside the trail, hands on their knees, catching their breath. At 1.9 miles, pass a cable that helps hikers negotiate ice in winter.

Soon you top out on the rib ridge of the Chimneys. ▶3 It extends from Sugarland Mountain, to your left. To your right are the twin peaks that reminded some pioneer long ago of a

Swimming

Stream

Steep

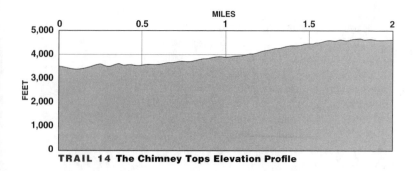

TRAIL 14 The Chimney Tops Elevation Profile

The rocky Chimney Tops *rise above Newfound Gap Road.*

chimney in a house. There actually is a hole in the rock, big enough to fall in. The native Cherokee, fancying the rock formation to be the branched horns of a deer, called this place Forked Antler. Be very careful as you climb up the open face rock, 4,755 feet high.

 Geologic Interest

To your east, beyond the second chimney, stands Mount Le Conte. To your west is the wooded wall of Sugarland Mountain. Southward stands Mount Mingus. To the north lies the valley of the West Prong of the Little Pigeon River and Newfound Gap Road, your return destination. The views here can be truly incredible.

 Photo Opportunity

 Great Views

🚶	MILESTONES	
▶1	0.0	Chimney Tops Trailhead
▶2	0.9	Road Prong Trail leaves left
▶3	2.0	The Chimney Tops

To Newfound Gap

Little River

Clingmans Dome Road

Clingmans Dome

Forney Ridge Trail

P

start & finish

Keeyuga Creek

Forney Creek

Kuwahi Branch

Spud Town Branch

Steeltrap Creek

Rattler Branch

Devil Branch

Snake Tongue

Grouse Creek

GREAT SMOKY MOUNTAINS NATIONAL PARK

Goshen Prong Trail

Double Springs Gap Shelter

Talassah Ridge

Higgins Creek

Goshen Prong

Spy Branch

Jenkins Knob

Little Higgins Creek

Suli Knob

Jonas Creek

TENNESSEE

NORTH CAROLINA

Narrows Branch

Silers Creek

Silers Bald

Silers Bald Shelter

Welch Ridge Trail

Lean-To Branch

0.75 miles

0.5

0.25

0.75 kilometers

0.5

0.25

0

N

Silers Bald via Clingmans Dome

Begin at the park's highest trailhead, near Clingmans Dome, and follow the Appalachian Trail along a knife-edge ridge. Roller-coaster along the spine of the Smokies, presenting stellar views. Reach the fast disappearing field of Silers Bald, enjoying multiple vistas.

Best Time

Clingmans Dome Road, the trail access and where this hike begins, is open from April through November. Spring and fall have the clearest skies for stupendous views. Summer is plenty cool, but can be stormy in the afternoons. If you want to camp, try to stay at Silers Bald during the week.

Finding the Trail

From Newfound Gap, drive 7 miles to the end of Clingmans Dome Road. The Forney Ridge Trail starts at the southwestern end of the Clingmans Dome parking area, where the road begins looping away from Clingmans Dome.

Trail Description

This hike fairly exudes the aura of the high country, as you traverse in and out of the spruce-fir forest that cloaks only the highest mantles of this land. Start your hike at the highest trailhead in the park, 6,400 feet, just below Clingmans Dome. Straddle the very spine of the state line ridge, joining the Appalachian Trail southbound. Enjoy all-encompassing windswept vistas into both states that

TRAIL USE
Dayhiking, Backpacking
LENGTH
9.6 miles, 5–6 hours
VERTICAL FEET
+1,200/-1,200
DIFFICULTY
– 1 2 **3** 4 5 +
TRAIL TYPE
Out & Back

FEATURES
Great Views
Ridgeline
Summit
Autumn Colors
Wildflowers
Spruce-fir
Photo Opportunity

FACILITIES
Restrooms
Water
Camping

comprise the Smoky Mountains. Culminate your hike on Silers Bald, where you can look back and see where you came from and will return.

Start your hike at the Clingmans Dome parking area, ▶1 leaving on the Forney Ridge Trail. Crowds mill about in summer, taking the short quarter-mile path up to the viewing tower atop Clingmans Dome. At 0.1 mile veer right on the Clingmans Dome Bypass Trail. The evergreen smells of the spruce-fir forest waft into your nostrils as you soon leave the crowds behind. Moderately climb to intersect the Appalachian Trail near Mount Buckley, elevation 6,500 at 0.6 mile.

Continue southbound on the AT, dropping through an old burned-over section. The lack of tree cover opens vistas as far as the clarity of the sky allows. Drop into a saddle to briefly ascend again, topping out at a rock outcrop. This stone makes a wonderful bench to look far into North Carolina.

Reenter spruce-fir forest, moving downward all the while. The woods are nearly always wet and cool here. The average high temperatures are warmest in July atop Clingmans Dome, and that high is only 65 degrees. It rains upward of 90 inches per year at these heights.

🌲 **Spruce–Fir**

🔺 **Ridgeline**

🔭 **Great Views**

TRAIL 15 Silers Bald via Clingmans Dome Elevation Profile

After a brief level section, come to the Goshen Prong Trail junction at 2.5 miles. ▶2 Continue your descent on the AT to arrive at Double Springs Gap trail shelter, elevation 5,507 feet at mile 3.1. ▶3 A small clearing stands in front of the shelter. The two springs here flow into Tennessee and North Carolina respectively. The spring to your left, in North Carolina, as you arrive at the shelter, is the easiest one to obtain water from.

Backcountry Camping

Leave the shelter behind and climb Jenkins Knob, jumbled with beech trees. Beech leaves turn brown and often stay on the tree throughout the winter, rattling in the wind. Below the knob you'll come to a declining field at mile 3.5. Welch Ridge lines the horizon as you look into North Carolina. Pass through the Narrows, where the state line ridge becomes barely wide enough for a footpath.

Meet the Welch Ridge Trail at mile 4.4. ▶4 Now it is time to climb. Begin the final push to arrive on top of Silers Bald, 5,607 feet, at mile 4.6. ▶5 Note the USGS survey marker embedded into rock. Look back at the rugged crest of the Smokies. A small side trail to your right as you arrive at Silers allows long views into Tennessee from a rock outcrop. To your left the AT continues down the nearly disappeared bald, which the park service is allowing to reforest, to the Silers Bald trail shelter ▶6 and a spring at 4.8 miles. This popular shelter remains a good destination.

 Summit

 Photo Opportunity

🚶	**MILESTONES**	
▶1	0.0	Clingmans Dome Trailhead
▶2	2.5	Goshen Prong Trail leaves right
▶3	3.1	Double Springs Gap Shelter
▶4	4.4	Welch Ridge Trail leaves left
▶5	4.6	Top of Silers Bald
▶6	4.8	Silers Bald Shelter

CHAPTER 3

Mount Le Conte, Greenbrier, and Cosby Area

Mount Le Conte, Greenbrier, and Cosby Area

The Mount Le Conte, Greenbrier, and Cosby area covers the most northeasterly part of the Tennessee Smokies. Mount Le Conte, the third highest peak in the park, stands alone, disjunct from the main mountain crest, and towers over the adjacent mountainscape from 6,593 feet. The state line ridge extends east from Newfound Gap and presents a long continuous stretch of spruce-fir highlands, with connecting ridges also sporting the Canadian-type woodland. Other prominent peaks include Greenbrier Pinnacle and Mount Cammerer, with its historic stone tower. The area is drained by mountaintop springs gathering force to become full-fledged streams, all flowing into the Little Pigeon and Pigeon Rivers outside the park. Elevations range from nearly 6,600 feet atop Le Conte and the Tennessee shoulder of Mount Guyot to just under 1,500 feet near the Greenbrier park entrance. This vertical variation leads to natural variety as well. The flora and fauna replicate a trip up the spine of the Appalachians, from Georgia to Maine, with a decided prominence of northern plants and animals.

Newfound Gap Road forms the western boundary of the area. It has trail accesses low and high, from Sugarlands Visitor Center to Newfound Gap. US 321 runs east-west along the north park boundary, linking Le Conte, Greenbrier, and Cosby. One-way in, one-way out roads pierce both Cosby and Greenbrier, providing trail access. TN 32 wanders along the most northeasterly park border and ends near North Carolina's Big Creek Ranger Station and campground.

Though the land was not conducive for it, the terrain was heavily settled in pre-park days. The Sugarlands, in the northern shadow of Le Conte, was full of hardscrabble subsistence farms. Greenbrier also reflects its past in numerous homesites, reduced to piled rock fences, crumbling chimneys, or

Overleaf and opposite: Mount LeConte *as seen from Charlies Bunion (Trail 16)*

rusting old washtubs. The subsistence lifeways of the pioneer can be found along most every streamside flat in Cosby, too. As abundant as were the valley-dwelling mountaineers, the looming high country was just as dark and wild. The evergreen mantle atop ol' Smoky was mostly trailless country then. Parts of it remain that way today.

The trail system reflects this pattern. Ridgetop paths, created after the park's inception, travel in dense woods perched atop sometimes knife-edge ridges. On the other hand, low-elevation streamside trails are rarely far from an old flat once claimed by an independent mountain man and his offspring.

Hikes in this area run the gamut, offering something for everyone, from high to low, from long to short, from easy strolls to rugged backpacks. The peak of Mount Le Conte is the nexus for trails that lace it from all sides. Paths here feature grand vistas, abundant waterfalls, history, and fascinating geology. Today, a primitive lodge and backpack shelter present overnight accommodations for those willing to climb to them. In Greenbrier, it is hard to hike without encountering pioneer history, yet it has superlative natural delights such as Ramsey Cascades, a cataract set amid old-growth woodlands. Likewise, Cosby has the ancient forest of Albright Grove, views from Maddron Bald and Mount Cammerer scattered amid a pioneer past.

Cosby has the area's only campground. It is large and alluring—it's puzzling why more park visitors don't use it as a basecamp. Picnic areas can be found at Greenbrier, Cosby, and Sugarlands. Civilization is a short drive away. Accommodations, restaurants, and more can be found along the non-park roads from Gatlinburg to I-40 and the locale's eastern access.

Permits

Permits are *not* required for dayhiking. Backpackers, however, must get a backcountry permit to stay at one of the 12 designated backcountry campsites and trail shelters located in this area. Some require a simple self-registration; however, most require a reservation, which you can make by calling the backcountry permit office at (865) 436-1231. Pick up and fill out backcountry permits at Greenbrier Ranger Station or the Cosby Campground entrance station. If you're traveling in the high country, obtain your permit at Oconaluftee Visitor Center when coming from North Carolina or the Sugarlands Visitor Center when coming from Tennessee.

A giant tulip tree *rises skyward at Albright Grove (Trail 22)*

Mount Le Conte, Greenbrier, and Cosby Area

TRAIL FEATURES TABLE

Mount Le Conte, Greenbrier, and Cosby Area

TRAIL	Difficulty	Length	Type	USES & ACCESS	TERRAIN	FLORA & FAUNA	OTHER
16	3–4	8.0	Point-to-Point	Dayhiking, Backpacking	Summit, Ridgeline	Spruce-fir	Great Views, Photo Opportunity, Geologic Interest
17	2–3	4.6	Point-to-Point	Dayhiking	Stream, Ridgeline	Autumn Colors, Wildlife, Old-growth	Great Views, Historic Interest, Geologic Interest
18	2–3	5.4	Point-to-Point	Dayhiking	Stream, Waterfall	Autumn Colors, Wildflowers, Old-growth	Geologic Interest
19	4	6.6	Point-to-Point	Dayhiking	Stream, Waterfall, Summit, Ridgeline	Autumn Colors, Wildflowers, Old-growth	Great Views, Photo Opportunity, Geologic Interest
20	2–3	6.4	Point-to-Point	Dayhiking, Backpacking	Stream, Ridgeline	Autumn Colors, Wildflowers	Secluded, Historic Interest
21	4	8.0	Point-to-Point	Dayhiking	Stream, Waterfall	Autumn Colors, Wildflowers, Old-growth	Swimming, Geologic Interest
22	3	6.7	Loop	Dayhiking	Stream	Autumn Colors, Wildflowers, Old-growth	Secluded, Historic Interest
23	4–5	17.3	Loop	Backpacking	Stream, Waterfall, Ridgeline	Autumn Colors, Wildflowers, Old-growth	Great Views
24	2	3.6	Point-to-Point	Dayhiking, Child Friendly	Stream, Ridgeline	Autumn Colors, Wildflowers	Great Views, Photo Opportunity, Historic Interest
25	5	11.2	Point-to-Point	Dayhiking	Stream, Summit, Ridgeline	Autumn Colors, Wildflowers	Great Views, Photo Opportunity, Historic Interest, Geologic Interest

Legend

USES & ACCESS	TYPE	TERRAIN	FLORA & FAUNA	FEATURES
Dayhiking	Loop	Mountain	Autumn Colors	Great Views
Backpacking	Out & Back	Summit	Wildflowers	Photo Opportunity
Horses	Point-to-Point	Ridgeline	Wildlife	Backcountry Camping
Child Friendly	DIFFICULTY -1 2 3 4 5 + less more	Stream	Spruce-fir	Swimming
		Waterfall	Old-growth	Secluded
		Lake		Steep
				Historic Interest
				Geologic Interest

Maps

For the Mount Le Conte, Greenbrier, and Cosby area, here are the USGS 7.5-minute (1:24,000-scale) topographic quadrangles that you will need, listed in the order that you will need them as you hike along your route.

Trail 16: Clingmans Dome, Mount Le Conte
Trail 17: Mount Le Conte
Trail 18: Mount Le Conte
Trail 19: Mount Le Conte
Trail 20: Mount Le Conte
Trail 21: Mount Guyot

Trail 22: Jones Cove, Mount Guyot
Trail 23: Hartford, Jones Cove, Mount Guyot, Luftee Knob
Trail 24: Hartford
Trail 25: Hartford, Luftee Knob

Mount Le Conte, Greenbrier, and Cosby Area

Brushy Mountain via Grotto Falls ... 141

This hike takes you to appropriately named Roaring Fork to reach Grotto Falls, a popular cascade. The crowds disappear as you climb to Trillium Gap. A short ramble leads atop Brushy Mountain, where views await amid a heath bald plant community.

TRAIL 19

Dayhiking
6.6 miles, Out & Back
Difficulty: 1 2 **3 4** 5

Injun Creek from Greenbrier 147

This secluded hike skirts the lower reaches of Mount Le Conte. Pass a collection of former farms and homesites dotting Greenbrier. End at the Injun Creek backcountry campsite, #32, just above which lies a wrecked steam engine tractor, a high-tech contraption that crashed before the park was established.

TRAIL 20

Dayhiking, Backpacking
6.4 miles, Out & Back
Difficulty: 1 **2 3** 4 5

Ramsey Cascades 153

This rewarding hike presents a waterfall and old-growth woodlands in a remote area of the park. Start out with a slight upgrade, then climb more steeply through old-growth trees in virgin woods as you near the cascades. The area remains as it has for ages.

TRAIL 21

Dayhiking
8.0 miles, Out & Back
Difficulty: 1 2 3 **4** 5

Albright Grove 157

Hike from a lesser-used trailhead, passing the well-preserved Willis Baxter Cabin. Travel amid more pioneer homesites in quiet stream valleys before entering the land of giant trees—old-growth forest now preserved forever. The uppermost part of the hike makes a short loop between Dunn Creek and Indian Camp Creek, taking you by trees that helped supporters make the case for establishing the Smoky Mountains National Park.

TRAIL 22

Dayhiking
6.7 miles, Loop
Difficulty: 1 2 **3** 4 5

TRAIL 23

Backpacking

17.3 miles, Loop

Difficulty: 1 2 3 **4 5**

Maddron Bald Loop 163

This is one of the best backpacking loops in the entire park! First, hike along the lower reaches of Gabes Mountain, passing Hen Wallow Falls and entering virgin woodland to camp at Sugar Cove. Next, head up Maddron Bald Trail, to Albright Grove, which contains some of the park's largest trees. Camp along resonant high country Otter Creek. Surmount Maddron Bald, which sports awe-inspiring views. Return via the rugged Snake Den Trail, where more vistas open on heath balds.

TRAIL 24

Dayhiking,

Child Friendly

3.6 miles, Out & Back

Difficulty: 1 **2** 3 4 5

Sutton Ridge Overlook 171

This hike to Sutton Ridge Overlook is ideal for families that want to get off the beaten path. The Lower Mount Cammerer Trail initially passes through former pioneer lands, long since forested, to reach a brook trout stream, then climbs a bit to reach Sutton Ridge. A spur trail leads to a great view of the surrounding area.

TRAIL 25

Dayhiking

11.2 miles, Out & Back

Difficulty: 1 2 3 4 **5**

Mount Cammerer via Low Gap 175

Revel at great views from a historic restored lookout tower. Leave Cosby Campground, and head up Cosby Creek valley through gorgeous woodland to the state line. Meet the Appalachian Trail at Low Gap. Cruise the state line to emerge at an outcrop and tower where the world falls away.

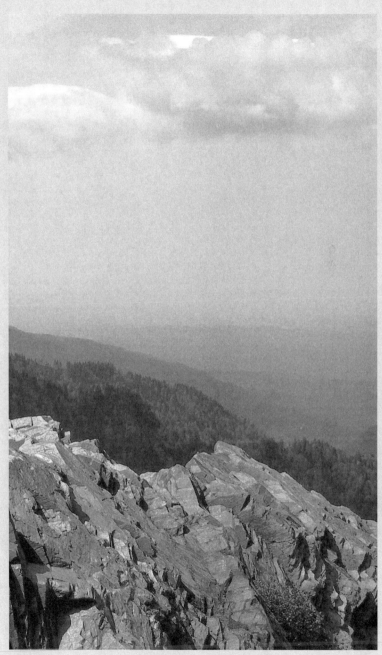

Charlies Bunion (*Trail 16*) *is a rocky crag perched above Porters Creek Valley.*

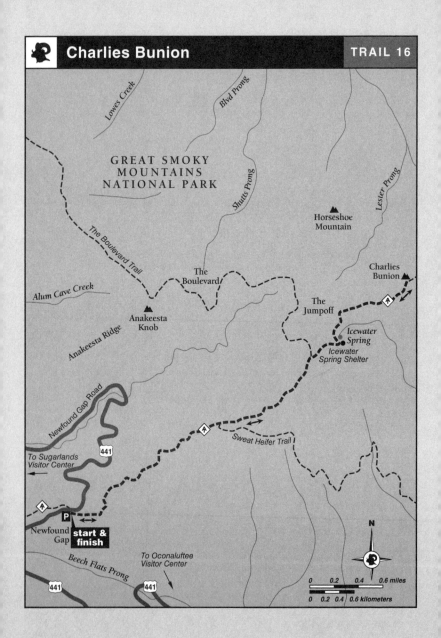

Charlies Bunion

TRAIL 16

GREAT SMOKY
MOUNTAINS
NATIONAL PARK

Lowes Creek

Blvd Prong

Shutts Prong

Lester Prong

Horseshoe
Mountain

The Boulevard Trail

Charlies
Bunion

The
Boulevard

The
Jumpoff

Alum Cave Creek

Anakeesta
Knob

Icewater
Spring

Anakeesta Ridge

Icewater
Spring Shelter

Newfound Gap Road

441

Sweat Heifer Trail

To Sugarlands
Visitor Center

Newfound
Gap

start & finish

P

N

To Oconaluftee
Visitor Center

Beech Flats Prong

441

441

0   0.2   0.4   0.6 miles

0   0.2   0.4   0.6 kilometers

Charlies Bunion

Leave busy Newfound Gap and head northbound on the Appalachian Trail. Rise amid rare spruce-fir forest with occasional clearings that present warm-up views. Pass Icewater Springs trail shelter before descending a knife-edge ridge. Come to the outcrop where amazing views into the Volunteer State and beyond open wide.

Best Time

The park tries to keep Newfound Gap Road open year-round; thus this trek is a good way to jump into the maw of a high country winter. Spring and fall are good choices with clear skies. Summer is busy.

Finding the Trail

From Tennessee's Sugarlands Visitor Center, drive 13.1 miles to Newfound Gap. The trailhead is on the parking area's left, near the large stone podium, with the plaque on it. From North Carolina's Oconaluftee Visitor Center, drive 16 miles to Newfound Gap. The trailhead is at the far end of the parking area as you come from the Tar Heel State.

Trail Description

The view from Charlies Bunion is arguably the park's finest. Unlike a view from a fire tower or a rounded peak, Charlies Bunion boasts a vista from a cliff face with an abrupt drop of more than 1,000 feet! But you will soak in fine views on your hike to

TRAIL USE
Dayhiking, Backpacking

LENGTH
8.0 miles, 4–5 hours

VERTICAL FEET
+1,500/-1,500

DIFFICULTY
– 1 2 **3 4** 5 +

TRAIL TYPE
Out & Back

FEATURES
Ridgeline
Summit
Spruce-fir
Great Views
Geologic Interest
Photo Opportunity

FACILITIES
Restrooms
Water

TRAIL 16 Charlies Bunion Elevation Profile

the bunion, interspersed with sections of spruce-fir high country forest.

Unusual for the timeworn Appalachian Range, the precipitous Charlies Bunion is the result of two events in the 1920s. A devastating fire raged over the area that is the bunion in 1925, denuding the vegetation clinging to the thin mountaintop soils. In 1929, heavy rains triggered a landslide of the burned-over area, leaving bare rock—and a great view—in its wake.

Head east from Newfound Gap ▶1 on possibly the most hiked quarter mile of the entire Appalachian Trail. As you climb away from the gap, the throngs soon disappear, turning around after getting a mild taste of America's most famous footpath. The trail is rocky and often wet, use caution. Spruce-fir woodlands flank the track. Continue to wind up the side of Mount Kephart, named for writer and early park proponent Horace Kephart. The southern flank of Mount Le Conte stands to your left.

The Appalachian Trail comes to a level area and the Sweat Heifer Trail junction at mile 1.7. ▶2 The trail is often muddy here as it passes the 6,000-foot mark only to descend to meet the Boulevard Trail at mile 2.7. ▶3 The Boulevard Trail links the main crest of the Appalachians to Mount Le Conte, and is

🌲 Spruce–Fir

🔺 Ridgeline

not nearly as easy as its name implies. Stay on the evergreen-flanked Appalachian Trail, opening up at the Icewater Springs trail shelter, at mile 2.9. ▶4 The revamped shelter is surrounded by a clearing and displays impressive views. Icewater Spring, with its well-deserved name, is just beyond the shelter.

Backcountry Camping

Beyond the spring, a half-mile decline on a rocky, wet slope leads to a narrow stretch of the main state line ridge. At mile 3.6 a good vista opens and you can see the rocky point of Charlies Bunion below. Arrive at a trail junction at mile 4.0, just before Charlies Bunion. The Appalachian Trail leaves right. Carefully follow the narrow trail 100 yards left to arrive at Charlies Bunion. ▶5

Great Views

Below you lies the remote Greenbrier area of the park. To your left rises Mount Le Conte. The green heath bald of Brushy Mountain is visible. A sunny clear day allows an unparalleled view into the hills of East Tennessee. At your feet, dark-eyed juncos and Eastern chipmunks vie for some of your trail mix. This is a great place to appreciate just how high the Smoky Mountains are, and how cataclysmic events can reveal their bedrock—and great views.

Photo Opportunity

Geologic Interest

🚶	**MILESTONES**	
▶1	0.0	Newfound Gap Trailhead
▶2	1.7	Sweat Heifer Trail leaves right
▶3	2.7	Boulevard Trail leaves left
▶4	2.9	Icewater Springs trail shelter
▶5	4.0	Charlies Bunion

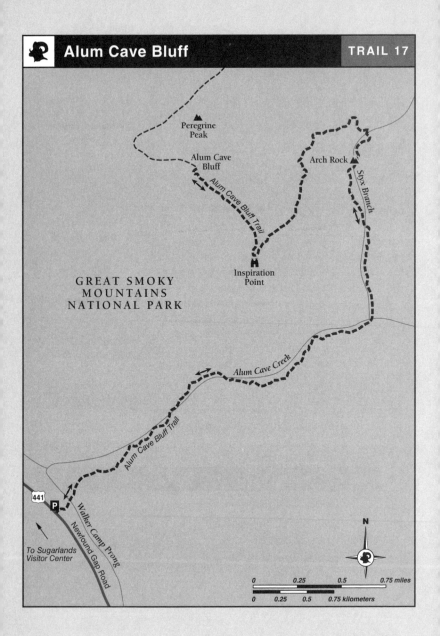

Peregrine
Peak

Alum Cave
Bluff

Arch Rock

Styx Branch

Alum Cave Bluff Trail

Inspiration
Point

GREAT SMOKY
MOUNTAINS
NATIONAL PARK

Alum Cave Creek

Alum Cave Bluff Trail

441

P

Walker Camp Prong

Newfound Gap Road

To Sugarlands
Visitor Center

N

| 0 | 0.25 | 0.5 | 0.75 miles |
| 0 | 0.25 | 0.5 | 0.75 kilometers |

Alum Cave Bluff

Some hikes are busy for a reason. This one has several, including highlights ranging from spectacular views to old-growth forests to a natural arch—rare for the Smokies—and finally to an overhanging bluff with views of its own. A well-timed hike will let you enjoy these highlights on a less-crowded trek.

Best Time

Winter offers the most solitude on this busy trek. Otherwise, try to hike early in the morning or later in the evening to avoid the crowds.

Finding the Trail

From the intersection of Newfound Gap Road and Little River Road near Sugarlands Visitor Center, drive 8.6 miles south on Newfound Gap Road to the Alum Cave Bluff parking area on your left.

Trail Description

The steep slopes of Mount Le Conte contain some of the most beautiful scenery in the Smokies. This hike travels an ancient forest along Alum Cave Creek before turning up Styx Branch, where Arch Rock awaits. This geological feature is different from other classic arches you may have seen; it is more of a circular maw, with stone steps leading through it. The hike then opens onto a heath bald where a rock promontory lives up to its name of Inspiration Point. Finally, climb a rock slope to reach Alum Cave Bluff, a huge rock overhang with views of its own.

TRAIL USE
Dayhiking
LENGTH
4.6 miles, 2–3 hours
VERTICAL FEET
+1,100/-1,100
DIFFICULTY
– 1 **2** 3 4 5 +
TRAIL TYPE
Out & Back

FEATURES
Stream
Ridgeline
Autumn Colors
Wildlife
Great Views
Old-growth
Geologic Interest
Historic Interest

FACILITIES
None

Try to hike during off-times to avoid the crowds. I suggest getting there at sunrise, during times when it may rain, or on winter weekdays. *Do not hike here during summer or holiday weekends,* as Smokies visitors sometimes clog this deserving highlight reel of a hike. It also gets use from folks hiking up and down on overnight trips to Mount Le Conte Lodge, closed during the winter.

Stream

Spur trails from the two large parking areas ►1 converge at the bridge over Walker Camp Prong, which you cross by footlog. Old-growth forest of yellow birch and spruce rise above the hiker-only trail as it slices through a rhododendron sea. Bridge Alum Cave Creek on a footlog. Notice that some of the hemlocks close to the trailhead are being preserved, but you will also see red spruce, another evergreen. Watch for a massive red spruce left of the trail at 0.4 mile. This is a good spot to look around

Old–growth

and take inventory of the ancient grove.

Authentic old-growth woodland is not an agglomeration of even-aged primeval trees. On the contrary, even aged trees are a result of disturbance. An old-growth forest has many big trees along with younger trees that grow when they get the chance. When a big tree falls, it creates a light gap. Young trees sprout in this light gap, and other partially

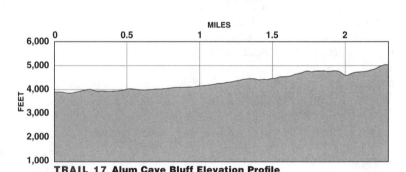

TRAIL 17 Alum Cave Bluff Elevation Profile

Alum Cave Bluff *overlooks the verdant forests of yon Smoky Mountains.*

mature trees thrive in the additional sun. Other times, in the dim of the dark forest, trees gain foothold on nurse logs.

Nurse logs (fallen and decaying trees) allow a seedling to gain root and then feed the young trees with the energy they contain. Later, the new trees grow and spread roots around the fallen log. Over time, a nurse log returns to the soil, and the newly grown tree looks as if it grew up with legs.

The heavily traveled trail has many exposed roots, so watch your footing as well as the stately giants above and the crystalline stream beside you, with its beige, gray, and tan rocks. Cross Alum Cave Creek on another footlog at mile 1.0. ▶2 The trail swerves left and begins to follow Styx Branch, which it bridges at 1.3 miles. Watch for a gigantic buckeye tree just after this crossing that brings you over to

Sand myrtle grows only along the Southeastern coastline and in the Southern Appalachians.

the left-hand bank. Next, come to one of nature's more time-consuming projects, Arch Rock, at 1.4 miles, ►3 just after another footlog crossing of Styx Branch.

Geologic Interest

At first, it seems that the path dead ends. However, a set of stone stairs leads the way through the tunnel-like arch. Continue ascending, stepping over Styx Branch a final time at 1.5 miles. Open

The great forests, which the Smokies are known for, cloak the lower slopes of Mount Le Conte.

onto an area (known as a heath bald) covered with small, low bushes. Rock outcrops are mixed among the low-slung Catawba rhododendron, sand myrtle, and mountain laurel, along with a few wind-sculpted trees.

Great views open from Inspiration Point at 2.0 miles. ▶4 See the Chimneys and Sugarland Mountain across the gulf, the rockslides of Anakeesta Ridge, and slides nearer to the west. Unstable soils have simply sloughed off the mountainside, usually following heavy rain. Give yourself ample time to relax at this superlative setting.

 Great Views

Leave the bald, cruising the rock face of Peregrine Peak, a stony knob of Mount Le Conte. Peregrine falcons were successfully reintroduced on Mount Le Conte. The mostly open rock trail can get quite icy in winter. The park service has strung wire handrails along the declivitous slope. Arrive at Alum Cave Bluff, residing at the 5,000-foot elevation, at 2.3 miles. ▶5 The rock overhang with a dusty floor really isn't a cave. During the Civil War, soldiers led by Chief Thomas Walker and his band of Confederate Cherokees mined the bluff for saltpeter to make gunpowder for the South. You can usually smell sulfur at the bluff. In the winter, large icicles form atop the overhang and crash down when the air warms. Nature is constantly at work on the Alum Cave Bluff Trail.

 Wildlife

 Geologic Interest

 Historic Interest

🚶	MILESTONES	
▶1	0.0	Alum Cave Trailhead
▶2	1.0	Cross Styx Branch
▶3	1.4	Arch Rock
▶4	2.0	Inspiration Point
▶5	2.3	Alum Cave Bluff

Rainbow Falls

TRAIL 18

Falls Branch

To
Gatlinburg

Roaring Fork Motor
Nature Trail

start &
finish
P

Cherokee Orchard Road

Trillium Gap Trail

Rocky Spur Branch

Old
Sugarlands
Trail

Rainbow Falls Trail

Le Conte Creek

GREAT SMOKY
MOUNTAINS
NATIONAL PARK

Le Conte Creek

Rainbow
Falls

Bullhead Trail

N

0   0.1   0.2   0.3 miles

0   0.1   0.2   0.3 kilometers

Rainbow Falls

This deservedly popular hike reaches a waterfall on the shoulder of Mount Le Conte. Hike up attractive Le Conte Creek Valley, where the creek cascades over rocks and into pools. Trek among big boulders and under old-growth trees to reach Rainbow Falls, a curtain-type cascade.

Best Time

The falls are their boldest in winter and spring. Wildflowers are abundant in spring also. Summer can be too crowded.

Finding the Trail

From Sugarlands Visitor Center, take US 441 into Gatlinburg and reach traffic light #8, Airport Road. Turn right on Airport Road and follow it 0.6 mile, then keep forward, joining Cherokee Orchard Road to enter the park. At 3.8 miles, reach the Rainbow Falls Trailhead, just after passing Old Sugarlands Trail.

Trail Description

There's no doubt about it—waterfalls attract hikers. They are a scenic destination, an endpoint that changes with the seasons. At Rainbow Falls, you may get a frozen curtain falling off the sheer rock face. In spring, the heavy flow may have a pile of melting ice under it. In summer, throngs trek through deep woods to the rock cathedral on the cool north side of Mount Le Conte. In fall, colorful

TRAIL USE
Dayhiking

LENGTH
5.4 miles, 3–4 hours

VERTICAL FEET
+1,650/-1,650

DIFFICULTY
– 1 **2 3** 4 5 +

TRAIL TYPE
Out & Back

FEATURES
Stream
Waterfall
Autumn Colors
Wildflowers
Old-growth
Geologic Interest

FACILITIES
Restrooms

trees flank hikers as they find a thin veil of water gently spilling over stone.

When the sun spills just right over the mist from the fall, a rainbow forms, giving the cataract its name. Leaving the main parking area, ▶1 cruising a wooded slope. Several user-created trails make this area potentially confusing. You will shortly end up at the intersection with the Trillium Gap Trail. ▶2 Stay with the Rainbow Falls Trail, soon coming alongside Le Conte Creek. This fast-moving rocky brook became known as Mill Creek because there were so many small-scale corn-grinding water-powered tub mills along its banks. It seems more rock than water as it bounds toward the town of Gatlinburg from the highlands of Mount Le Conte. Overhead red maples, oaks, black birches, and a scattering of preserved hemlocks shade the trail. The well-beaten root-covered track is scattered with gravel. Spur paths lead to the boisterous creek.

Keep uphill and upstream in the wildflower- and rhododendron-filled valley. At 0.5 mile, the trail switchbacks then turns back up the valley. Come alongside Le Conte Creek at 0.9 mile, only to turn away again, joining a drier slope with galax, mountain laurel, and chestnut oaks. At 1.1 miles, on another switchback, an obscured view extends toward Gatlinburg. The path then passes some big

 Stream

 Autumn Colors

Wildflowers

TRAIL 18 Rainbow Falls Elevation Profile

boulders upon which hikers scramble. A small overhang could provide shelter from a thunderstorm.

 Geologic Interest

The Rainbow Falls Trail works into the valley
again, coming alongside Le Conte Creek at 1.6
miles. Cooler climate trees, such as yellow birch and
cherry, show a presence. Look also for big preserved
hemlocks. At 1.8 miles, cross Le Conte Creek on a
footbridge. ▶3 Take in creek views here at nearly
3,700 feet. Enter a world of big trees, passing a
massive hemlock on trail right at 1.9 miles. ▶4 Start
switchbacking up a rich, mossy slope between Le
Conte Creek and a tributary, avoiding the shortcuts
used by thoughtless hikers.

Old–growth

At 2.3 miles, the trail reaches a tributary just
below a small waterfall, a preview of your destination. Rock-hop the tributary. ▶5 Come back
alongside Le Conte Creek at 2.5 miles, then bridge
it at 2.6 miles. ▶6 The trail leads farther up and
to another bridge. You are there! Uphill, beyond a
boulder field, spills Rainbow Falls. ▶7 The stream
tumbles 80 feet over a wide stone face into a rocky
cathedral. You must do a little boulder scrambling
to get close to the falls. Be careful as the rocks are
often slick. A good view can be had from the trail.

Waterfall

On your way back—if the trail is busy—count
how many hikers ask you, "How much farther?"
This path seems to attract hikers with more desire
than stamina to make the 1,600-foot climb.

🚶	MILESTONES	
▶1	0.0	Rainbow Falls Trailhead
▶2	0.1	Stay straight as Trillium Gap Trail leaves left
▶3	1.8	Bridge Le Conte Creek
▶4	1.9	Huge hemlock
▶5	2.3	Rock-hop tributary below fall
▶6	2.6	Bridge Le Conte Creek
▶7	2.7	Rainbow Falls

Mount
Winnesoka

Lookout Rock

Roaring Fork

Rocky Spur Branch

Roaring Fork Motor Nature Trail

Enloe Hollow Branch

Long Branch
Gap

P

**start &
finish**

Trillium Gap Trail

Surry Fork

Brushy
Mountain

Grotto
Falls

Trillium
Gap

Trillium Gap Trail

Brushy
Mountain Trail

Trillium
Branch

Roaring Fork

GREAT SMOKY
MOUNTAINS
NATIONAL PARK

Rainbow
Falls

Rocky Spur

Le Conte Creek

N

0   0.1   0.2   0.3 miles

0   0.1   0.2   0.3 kilometers

Brushy Mountain via Grotto Falls

This hike takes you to appropriately named Roaring Fork to reach Grotto Falls, a popular cascade. The crowds disappear as you climb to Trillium Gap. A short ramble leads atop Brushy Mountain, where views await amid a heath bald plant community.

Best Time

Roaring Fork Motor Nature Trail is generally closed from late November until mid-March, cutting off trailhead access. In spring Grotto Falls are bold, and the views from Brushy Mountain are extensive. During warmer times the trail to Grotto Falls can be crowded. Fall is a good choice, with clear skies presenting far-reaching panoramas.

Finding the Trail

From Sugarlands Visitor Center, take US 441 into Gatlinburg and reach traffic light #8, Airport Road. Turn right on Airport Road and follow it 0.6 mile, then keep forward, joining Cherokee Orchard Road to enter the park. At 4 miles, reach the Roaring Fork Motor Nature Trail. Turn right here and follow the one-way road 1.7 miles to the Trillium Gap connector access on your right, just as the motor trail makes a hard left.

Trail Description

This trek is a tale of two hikes. Down low you have water and crowds, while up high you enjoy solitude and vistas—all on the same hike. The first

TRAIL USE
Dayhiking

LENGTH
6.6 miles, 3–4 hours

VERTICAL FEET
+1,680/-1,680

DIFFICULTY
- 1 2 **3 4** 5 +

TRAIL TYPE
Out & Back

FEATURES
Ridgeline
Stream
Summit
Old-growth
Waterfall
Autumn Colors
Wildflowers
Great Views
Geologic Interest
Photo Opportunity

FACILITIES
None

> Stop to absorb
> the ambiance of
> this place with its
> perpetual cool breeze
> under whispering
> beech trees.

Old-growth

Stream

part travels to Grotto Falls, an interesting cascade that tumbles over a deep rock overhang. You actually walk behind and under the falls on the way to Trillium Gap Trail. This part of the trail can be very crowded, but beyond Grotto Falls the pathway is likely to be deserted.

You then climb into northern hardwoods mixed with spruce to reach Trillium Gap. From here the path cuts into an evergreen heath bald atop, which has extensive panoramas of the Smokies and the nearby lands that border it. For an easy family hike, just walk to Grotto Falls and back.

Take the well-used connector path ▶1 leading to the Trillium Gap Trail, upward among preserved hemlocks, many of them old-growth. Carolina silverbell, black birch, and yellow birch also line the rocky, root-covered track. Continue along a stream then reach a trail junction at 0.2 mile. ▶2 Turn left here joining the Trillium Gap Trail.

Step over a tributary and keep working your way between ridges and little hollows on the side of Mount Le Conte. The cool, north-facing slope harbors ferns, doghobble, and buckeye. Cross another small branch at 0.6 mile. You may notice more hemlocks aren't being preserved than are. Skeletal trunks rise in the forest. Step over another branch at 0.9 mile, and another at 1.0 mile.

TRAIL 19 Brushy Mountain via Grotto Falls Elevation Profile

Curve into Roaring Fork valley at 1.1 miles. Saddle up to the mountain cataract. Watch for a preliminary 15-foot two-tiered waterfall. It splits between two big boulders and forms a big pool below. The open rock face atop this fall beckons trailside relaxers.

Waterfall

You reach Grotto Falls at 1.4 miles. ▶3 Roaring Fork dives into a plunge pool around which hikers gather. Then you see people walking behind the falls.

Photo Opportunity

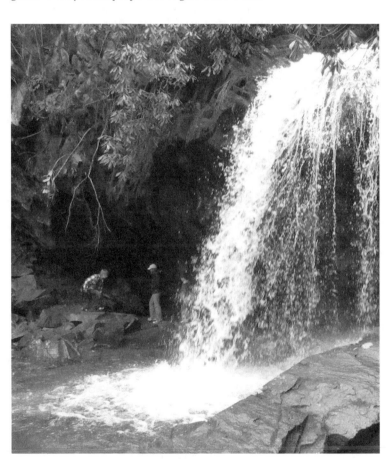

Hikers walk *through the overhang at Grotto Falls.*

The overhang behind the falls is how the cascade gets its name. It is fun to walk behind the spilling water, the official track.

Cruise behind the falls and continue up the Trillium Gap Trail. The crowds drop to your average backcountry trail, rather than those you find on an easy waterfall hike. Step over a trickling branch at 2.0 miles. You have broken the 4,000-foot elevation barrier. A few spruce trees appear among the northern hardwoods. Big boulders and rock fields border the path. Mosses and ferns find purchase on these trailside boulders. Pass a craggy, rock bluff at 2.4 miles. ▶4 At 2.5 miles, rock-hop Surry Fork, your last water source.

 Geologic Interest

The woodland understory becomes grassier as you approach Trillium Gap. Reach the gap at 3.0 miles. ▶5

To reach the top of Brushy Mountain, veer left from the gap and follow the path tunneling bushy evergreens. At 3.3 miles, you come to trail's end. ▶6

 Great Views

Viewpoints diverge from the main trail. Brushy Mountain offers panoramas both above and below your 4,900-foot elevation. Above and to your south stands the imposing bulk of Mount Le Conte. To your east, lies the Porters Creek valley. Below, to the north, stretches Gatlinburg and East Tennessee.

 Photo Opportunity

Heath Balds

FLORA

Heath balds form an interesting plant community in the Southern Appalachians. Generally treeless, they are concentrations of plants found on high ridges. The plants, including azaleas, blueberries, and sand myrtle, along with rhododendron and mountain laurel, grow in wind-sculpted tight thickets that native mountaineers dubbed "hells," since they were "hell to get into, and hell to get out of." Their origin is about as unclear as grassy balds, though exposure, soils, and fire are thought to play a role in their evolution.

🚶	**MILESTONES**	
▶1	0.0	Trillium Gap Trail Connector
▶2	0.2	Left on Trillium Gap Trail
▶3	1.4	Grotto Falls
▶4	2.4	Craggy bluff
▶5	3.0	Trillium Gap
▶6	3.3	Brushy Mountain

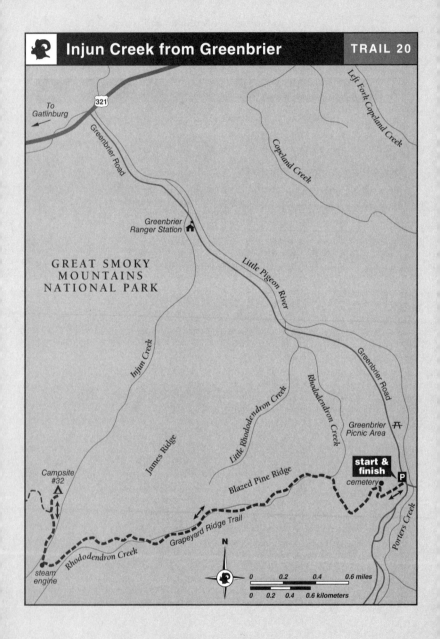

Injun Creek from Greenbrier — TRAIL 20

To Gatlinburg

321

Greenbrier Road

Greenbrier Ranger Station

GREAT SMOKY MOUNTAINS NATIONAL PARK

Little Pigeon River

Copeland Creek

Left Fork Copeland Creek

Greenbrier Road

Injun Creek

James Ridge

Little Rhododendron Creek

Rhododendron Creek

Greenbrier Picnic Area

start & finish

P

cemetery

Campsite #32

Blazed Pine Ridge

Grapeyard Ridge Trail

Porters Creek

steam engine

Rhododendron Creek

N

0   0.2   0.4   0.6 miles

0   0.2   0.4   0.6 kilometers

Injun Creek from Greenbrier

This secluded hike skirts the lower reaches of Mount Le Conte. Pass a collection of former farms and homesites dotting Greenbrier. End at the Injun Creek backcountry campsite, #32, just above which lies a wrecked steam engine tractor, a high-tech contraption that crashed before the park was established.

Best Time

Hikers heading here in fall will have the easiest stream crossings and the driest trail. Wildflowers are abundant in spring. Winter is a good time to see the plentiful trailside homesites. Summer could be warm.

Finding the Trail

From traffic light #3 on US 441 in Gatlinburg, take US 321, East Parkway, for 6.1 miles to the Greenbrier section of the park. Turn right and drive up Greenbrier Road for 3.1 miles to the intersection with Ramsey Prong Road, which crosses a bridge to your left. Park just before the intersection. The Grapeyard Ridge Trail starts on the right side of Greenbrier Road.

Trail Description

Greenbrier was one of the most heavily settled areas of what was to become Great Smoky Mountains National Park. Located in the shadow of Mount Le Conte, the rocky, mountainous area drains slopes

TRAIL USE
Dayhiking, Backpacking
LENGTH
6.4 miles, 3–4 hours
VERTICAL FEET
+850/-850
DIFFICULTY
– 1 **2 3** 4 5 +
TRAIL TYPE
Out & Back

FEATURES
Ridgeline
Stream
Autumn Colors
Wildflowers
Secluded
Historic Interest

FACILITIES
None

that flow north toward Gatlinburg and Pittman Center. The land is hardly arable, but mountain pioneers scraped out a living along the creek bottoms and sloped tributaries. This hike travels past several homesites located along Rhododendron Creek, a pleasant stream. You will become very familiar with the creek during several creek crossings as Grapeyard Ridge Trail seeks James Gap. From there you descend into the Injun Creek watershed.

The old farm turned backcountry campsite where you end the trek makes a great picnic or camping spot. Pull up a rock under the shade of a tree or simply sprawl out on the grass and contemplate what it might have been like to live here without the electrical accoutrements that accompany us through modern life.

Start the Grapeyard Ridge Trail on a Civilian Conservation Corps–built path ►1 that cobbles together old roads used by area settlers, passing rock walls and other wagon tracks splintering off the one you're following. At 0.3 mile, on a left-turning switchback, a spur path leads right to a pioneer cemetery. Mixed woodland of sweetgum, holly, maple, and pine form the forest.

Ascend to a gap and the remnants of a homesite chimney at 0.6 mile. ►2 The dull roar of Middle

Historic Interest

Autumn Colors

TRAIL 20 Injun Creek from Greenbrier Elevation Profile

Prong Little Pigeon River fades. The trail follows a small rill to Rhododendron Creek in a young spindly forest that was open land fourscore past. At 0.8 mile, step over the small rill and enter a persistent field. Make the first of several crossings of Rhododendron Creek and its tributaries, none of **▶ Stream** which are deep, though you may wet your shoes a bit in winter or after heavy rains.

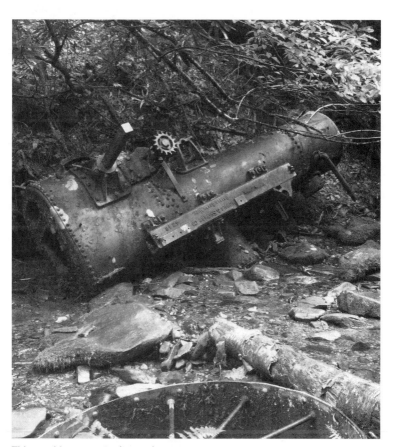

This machine *gave a Smokies creek a name.*

Historic Interest

Wildflowers

Autumn Colors

Ridgeline

Historic Interest

Backcountry Camping

Wind up the creek valley, noting the homesites on both sides of the path. Watch for exposed trailside white quartz. A 1931 topographic map of the Smokies, commissioned by the Department of the Interior, shows 11 homes in the Rhododendron Creek watershed. Watch for more closing fields in stream bottoms, which contrast greatly with the numerous rhododendron tunnels you pass through.

At 1.8 miles, a rock marks a spur trail leading left to a confusing network of old roads leading to forgotten homesites and graves of settlers who left the Smokies after it became a park. Down-trail, see where stones line the creek, marking a pioneer's attempt to tame Rhododendron Creek. Farmers in this rocky land couldn't afford to lose precious topsoil to sporadic flash floods that flushed the valley.

At 2.1 miles, leave Rhododendron Creek ►3 and begin the steady ascent to James Gap. A green cornucopia of rhododendron, mountain laurel, moss, and galax flank the path. Oaks and hickories stand overhead and drop their mast on the trail in fall. Another homesite, marked with a mere pile of rock rubble, sits in the saddle of James Gap at 2.8 miles. ►4 Enter the Injun Creek watershed. As you descend the inspiration for the creek's name appears in a rivulet on your right. The body and wheels of a tractorlike steam engine stand upturned, with water running beneath them. Somewhere in the naming of this creek an errant mapmaker thought the name referred to the Cherokee that roamed this land long ago and not a steam engine that made its final turn in the Great Smoky Mountains.

The old road-turned-trail descends to reach the spur path to Injun Creek backcountry campsite, #32. ►5 Turn right on the side trail to reach the camp at 3.2 miles. Enter yet another homesite. Walk around and look at the lasting changes the settlers made on the land, such as leveling the ground with rock walls. The campsite makes for a good break spot. On your return journey visualize this area in the future as the forest continues reestablishing its dominion over the Smokies.

🚶	MILESTONES	
▶1	0.0	Grapeyard Ridge Trailhead
▶2	0.6	Gap and homesite
▶3	2.1	Leave Rhododendron Creek
▶4	2.8	James Gap
▶5	3.2	Injun Creek campsite, #32

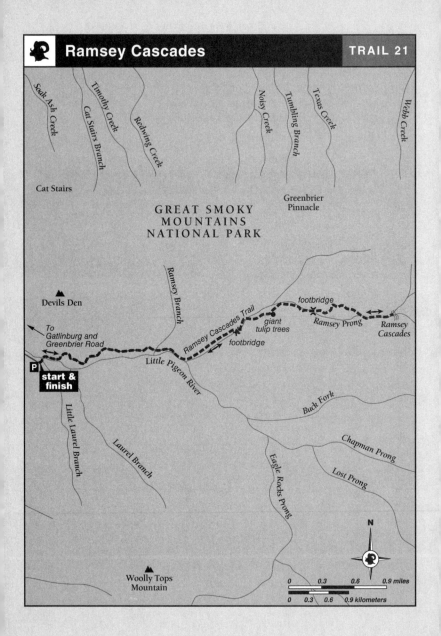

Soak Ash Creek

Timothy Creek

Cat Stairs Branch

Redwing Creek

Noisy Creek

Tumbling Branch

Texas Creek

Webb Creek

Cat Stairs

Greenbrier
Pinnacle

GREAT SMOKY
MOUNTAINS
NATIONAL PARK

Ramsey Branch

Devils Den

footbridge

Ramsey Cascades Trail

giant
tulip trees

Ramsey Prong

Ramsey
Cascades

To
Gatlinburg and
Greenbrier Road

footbridge

Little Pigeon River

P

**start &
finish**

Buck Fork

Little Laurel Branch

Laurel Branch

Eagle Rocks Prong

Chapman Prong

Lost Prong

N

Woolly Tops
Mountain

| 0 | 0.3 | 0.6 | 0.9 miles |
| 0 | 0.3 | 0.6 | 0.9 kilometers |

Ramsey Cascades

This rewarding hike presents a waterfall and old-growth woodlands in a remote area of the park. Start out with a slight upgrade, then climb more steeply through old-growth trees in virgin woods as you near the cascades. The area remains as it has been for ages.

TRAIL USE
Dayhiking

LENGTH
8.0 miles, 4½–5½ hours

VERTICAL FEET
+2,250/-2,250

DIFFICULTY
− 1 2 3 **4** 5 +

TRAIL TYPE
Out & Back

FEATURES
Stream
Waterfall
Old-growth
Geologic Interest
Autumn Colors
Wildflowers
Swimming

FACILITIES
None

Best Time

This hike is good year-round. However, spring has a plethora of wildflowers. Hikers can swim in summer. Fall has brilliant old-growth forests. In winter, Ramsey Cascades may be frozen, which attracts hikers, too.

Finding the Trail

From traffic light #3 on US 441 in Gatlinburg, take US 321, East Parkway, for 6.1 miles to the Greenbrier section of the park. Turn right and drive up Greenbrier Road for 3.1 miles to the intersection with Ramsey Prong Road, which crosses a bridge to your left. Turn left onto Ramsey Prong Road, crossing the road bridge, then follow the road 1.5 miles to dead end at the trailhead.

Trail Description

The hike leaves the trailhead, ▶1 passing around boulders. The Middle Prong Little Pigeon River crashes through the valley amid huge gray boulders and thousands of smaller rocks, sometimes slowing into ultraclear pools, sometimes sliding around

Stream

Geologic Interest

_____

**This is the valley
of the big trees:
tulip trees, Carolina
silverbells, buckeyes,
and more.**

_____

Old–growth

tree-covered islands, but always moving downstream. Soon cross the prong on a very long footbridge. The river is wide here. Stop for a moment and look upstream and downstream at this watercourse shaded in sycamores, birch, and rhododendron.

The wide track continues up the west side of Middle Prong. Huge boulders litter the mountainside. At 0.3 mile, a gigantic boulder forms a rock shelter. Climb away from the stream. Level off at 0.8 mile. Keep east in rocky terrain. Bridge Ramsey Branch at 1.3 miles, flowing down from Greenbrier Pinnacle, shading the trail to your left. At 1.5 miles, the trail comes to an old auto turnaround. ▶2 The Ramsey Cascade Trail continues straight, and climbs more steeply as it enters smaller and narrower Ramsey Prong Valley.

The trail morphs into a primitive footpath as it tunnels under rhododendron, climbing more steeply. Cross Ramsey Prong on a footlog at 2.1 miles. ▶3 Note the shaded pool below a rock overhang just below the bridge. That swimming hole stays chilly year-round!

At 2.5 miles, pass between two massive tulip trees that act as trailside gates, leading to a third tulip tree—the biggest of them all. ▶4 Impressive! At 2.8 miles, stone steps lead past a small rock shelter on trail right.

TRAIL 21 Ramsay Cascades Elevation Profile

Span Ramsey Prong yet again on a footlog at 3.0 miles. ▶5 Exposed roots over the people-worn path can make the trail tricky, especially while you're looking around at all the big trees. Now the path works left, crisscrossing a trickling tributary as it wanders through a cove full of big buckeyes and cherry trees. Return to Ramsey Prong at 3.6 miles. Keep ascending amid a mosaic of moss, boulders, birches, and rhododendron.

 Wildflowers

Rock-hop a tributary just before reaching the falls. Plunging down the green valley, nestled at 4,300 feet in elevation, between the high ridges of Guyot Spur and Pinnacle Lead, falls Ramsey Cascade, at mile 4.0. ▶6 Here, Ramsey Prong tumbles in a series of stair-step drops, framed by evergreens. Though it falls fewer than 100 feet, the cascade sends out quite a spray, which freezes in winter. Note the spruce trees, indicating your elevation. Picnickers and trail-weary hikers flock to the ample big boulders to watch this natural water show.

Waterfall

🚶	**MILESTONES**	
▶1	0.0	Ramsey Cascades Trailhead
▶2	1.5	Old auto turnaround
▶3	2.1	Bridge Ramsey Prong
▶4	2.5	Giant tulip trees
▶5	3.0	Bridge Ramsey Prong
▶6	4.0	Ramsey Cascades

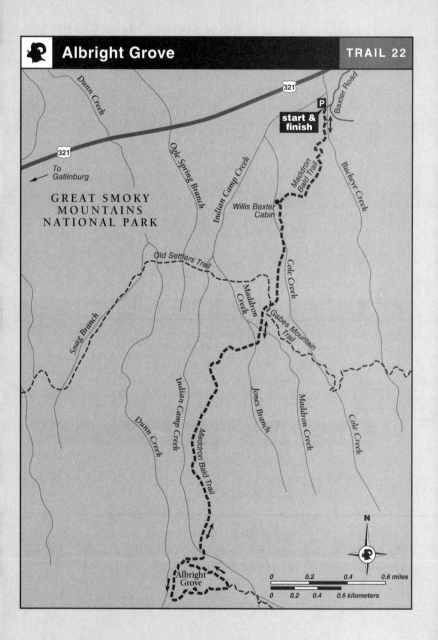

Albright Grove

TRAIL 22

321

start & finish

Baxter Road

Dunn Creek

321

To Gatlinburg

GREAT SMOKY MOUNTAINS NATIONAL PARK

Ogle Spring Branch

Indian Camp Creek

Willis Baxter Cabin

Maddron Bald Trail

Buckeye Creek

Cole Creek

Old Settlers Trail

Maddron Creek

Gabes Mountain Trail

Snag Branch

Dunn Creek

Indian Camp Creek

Maddron Bald Trail

Jones Branch

Maddron Creek

Cole Creek

Albright Grove

N

| 0 | 0.2 | 0.4 | 0.6 miles |

| 0 | 0.2 | 0.4 | 0.6 kilometers |

Albright Grove

Hike from a lesser-used trailhead, passing the well-preserved Willis Baxter Cabin. Travel amid more pioneer homesites in quiet stream valleys before entering the land of giant trees—old-growth forest now preserved forever. The uppermost part of the hike makes a short loop between Dunn Creek and Indian Camp Creek, taking you by trees that helped supporters make the case for establishing the Smoky Mountains National Park.

Best Time

During fall you will see not merely big trees but big trees cloaked in autumn finery. After the leaves have fallen, the many pioneer homesites of the area are more evident, as are big trees beyond the edge of the trail. This area is also a fine spring wildflower destination. Winter offers maximum seclusion.

Finding the Trail

From traffic light #3 in Gatlinburg, take US 321, East Parkway, north for 15.6 miles to Baxter Road, which is just beyond Jellystone Park Campground. Turn right onto Baxter Road and follow it for 0.3 mile to Laurel Springs Road. Veer sharply right onto the gravel Laurel Springs Road and follow it for 100 yards to a pole gate and trail sign on the left. The Maddron Bald Trail starts here.

TRAIL USE
Dayhiking
LENGTH
6.7 miles, 3–3½ hours
VERTICAL FEET
+1,500/-1,500
DIFFICULTY
– 1 2 **3** 4 5 +
TRAIL TYPE
Loop

FEATURES
Stream
Old-growth
Autumn Colors
Wildflowers
Secluded
Historic Interest

FACILITIES
None

Trail Description

A hard-to-find trailhead keeps many hikers off this trail. However, with good directions, it's a cinch. After finding the starting point, head up a wide bed on the Maddron Bald Trail. Pass the Willis Baxter Cabin, still intact after more than a century. Pass through a trail junction and start to climb a bit, then reach the side trail into Albright Grove. This nature trail loops through a giant forest of hemlock and tulip trees located between Dunn and Indian Camp Creeks. The immensity of this woodland, named after a former director of the park service, Horace Albright, makes this a trek that you will want to share with your friends.

The Maddron Bald Trail starts by passing a pole gate. ▶1 Buckeye Creek rushes downstream left of the trail. Head up an open roadbed beneath a second-growth deciduous forest, once farmland. Remember the size of these trees so that you can compare them to the big trees to come. The trail curves right toward Cole Creek and levels off, reaching the Willis Baxter Cabin at 0.6 mile. ▶2

 Historic Interest This one-room cabin was built in 1889. Note the notched logs at the cabin corners. There is a small

TRAIL 22 Albright Grove Elevation Profile

rocked-in spring and rock walls nearby. Developed springs are almost always found near old pioneer cabins and homesites.

Keep up Maddron Bald Trail, bridging Cole Creek, then reach a trail junction at 1.2 miles. ▶3 Gabes Mountain Trail leaves left to Cosby, and Old Settlers Trail leaves right to Greenbrier. History buffs can make a little side trip down Old Settlers Trail to see more homesites. Maddron Bald Trail

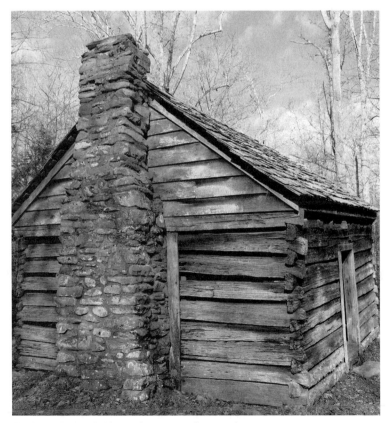

The Willis Baxter Cabin *stands against a pale winter sky.*

Stream

Old-growth

Some of these trees, such as Carolina silverbell and Fraser magnolia, are giants for their species.

Old-growth

slices between boulders and narrows, slipping over Maddron Creek and Jones Branch, which flow beneath the Civilian Conservation Corps–built trail. The path then passes through a small gap and drifts into the Indian Camp Creek streamshed. Indian Camp Creek dutifully roars in the lowlands below. The valley floor reveals rock walls and other trailside pioneer signs.

Reach an old auto turnaround at 2.3 miles. The path narrows yet again as it leaves the turnaround and the former civilized world. Big trees, primarily preserved hemlocks, immediately tower overhead. Come to Indian Camp Creek at 2.8 miles. ▶4 A long footbridge avails a dry footed crossing. Ascend steeply away from the creek, passing a seeping rock face that flows over the trail. The trail heads toward Dunn Creek before reaching a trail junction at 2.9 miles. ▶5

Stay forward with the Albright Grove Loop Trail, entering a sheltered valley with Indian Camp Creek to the east and Dunn Creek to the west. The north-facing slope ranges between 3,100 and 3,400 feet, ideal conditions for a Southern Appalachian cove hardwood forest. Deep, rich, and moist soils harbor not only massive trees but one of the temperate climate's most diverse plant communities overall. The dominant trees are hemlock, buckeye, Carolina silverbell, tulip trees, beech trees, yellow birch, and more. The list of smaller plants and herbs of the cove hardwood forest is long enough to numb a biologist.

Dunn Creek is audible through the rhododendron near the trail. Yellow birch trees shade mossy rocks and ferns. Turn away from Dunn Creek and climb along a hillside. A short path leads left to a tulip tree that has been towering since before the United States was established. Curve into a cove where buckeye trees dominate. From this cove the Albright Grove Nature Trail climbs to a ridgetop flat where hikers repose in the forest.

The tree grove was named for Horace Albright, the second director of the National Park Service. He was a big proponent of a national park for the Smokies, thinking that national parks should be well distributed throughout the country.

The Albright Grove Loop Trail then heads up the ridge nose. Cruise along a hillside with downward views toward Indian Camp Creek. Just before reaching the end of the trail, a massive barkless dead tree stands firm, despite being broken off 20 feet from its base. This tree, whatever it was, must've made quite a sound when it fell in the woods, even if no one was here to hear it.

The loop ends at 3.6 miles, ▶6 meeting the Maddron Bald Trail once again. From here, it is 0.3 mile back down to the lower end of the Albright Grove Loop Trail, ▶7 and a 2.9-mile backtrack to the Maddron Bald Trailhead. ▶8

Horace Albright successfully fought a mountain road that would have traversed the Smokies crest, similar to Skyline Drive at Shenandoah National Park.

🚶	MILESTONES	
▶1	0.0	Maddron Bald Trailhead
▶2	0.6	Willis Baxter Cabin
▶3	1.2	Old Settlers Trail and Gabes Mountain Trail
▶4	2.8	Bridge Indian Camp Creek
▶5	2.9	Right on Albright Grove Nature Trail
▶6	3.6	Left on Maddron Bald Trail
▶7	3.9	Meet lower end of Albright Grove Loop Trail and backtrack
▶8	6.7	Maddron Bald Trailhead

Maddron Bald Loop

TRAIL 23

GREAT SMOKY
MOUNTAINS
NATIONAL PARK

Caney Creek

Caney Creek Road

To
Gatlinburg

321

32

Cosby Creek

Big Branch

32

Riding Fork

Indian Camp Creek

Greenbrier Creek

Hen Wallow Creek

Crying Creek

Cosby Park Road

321

Willis Baxter
Cabin

Old Settlers
Trail

Buckeye Creek

Hen Wallow
Falls

Gabes Mountain Trail

**start &
finish**

P

Gabes Mountain Trail

Campsite
#34

Gabes Creek

Crying Creek

Cosby
Campground

cemetery

Jones Branch

Maddron Bald Trail

Indian Camp Creek

Dunn Creek

Cole Creek

Greenbrier Creek

Snake Den Ridge Trail

Inadu Creek

Little Rock Creek

Rock Creek

Camel Hump
Creek

Otter Creek

Albright
Grove

Maddron
Bald Trail

Campsite
#29

Copperhead
Branch

Big Creek

N

0   0.25   0.5   0.75 miles

0   0.25 0.5 0.75 kilometers

Maddron Bald Loop

This is one of the best backpacking loops in the entire park! First, hike along the lower reaches of Gabes Mountain, passing Hen Wallow Falls and entering virgin woodland to camp at Sugar Cove. Next, head up Maddron Bald Trail, to Albright Grove, which contains some of the park's largest trees. Camp along resonant high country Otter Creek. Surmount Maddron Bald, which sports awe-inspiring views. Return via the rugged Snake Den Trail, where more vistas open on heath balds.

Best Time

This destination is good year-round, though winter can be cold and harsh up high. The multiple creek crossings may be high in spring. High-elevation streamside camps are cool, even in summer. Fall offers low water and clear skies.

Finding the Trail

From Gatlinburg, take US 321 east until it comes to a T-intersection with TN 32. Follow TN 32 a little more than a mile, turning right into the signed Cosby section of the park. After 1.9 miles up Cosby Road, watch for a road splitting left to the picnic area. Turn left here and immediately park. The Gabes Mountain Trail starts a short distance downhill, back toward the entrance to Cosby, on the west side of Cosby Road.

TRAIL USE
Backpacking
LENGTH
17.3 miles, 6 hours
VERTICAL FEET
+4,000/-4,000
DIFFICULTY
- 1 2 3 **4 5** +
TRAIL TYPE
Loop

FEATURES
Stream
Ridgeline
Waterfall
Old-growth
Autumn Colors
Wildflowers
Great Views

SEASONAL FACILITIES
Water
Restrooms
Picnic area
Campground

Trail Description

Join the Gabes Mountain Trail ►1 just downhill from the Cosby picnic area. Dayhikers can make the trip to Hen Wallow Falls for a 4.4-mile rewarding trek round-trip. Pine, oak, and hickory forest bordered by rhododendron and mountain laurel shades the track. Reach a trail junction at 0.3 mile. A spur trail leads left to Cosby Campground. Stay right here to bridge Rock Creek. Step over streamlets flowing from Snake Den Mountain. More substantial tributaries have small bridges. Bridge Crying Creek before coming to an old auto turnaround at 1.1 miles. Climb past an old homestead—look for rocks piled in a vain attempt to make this hardscrabble, sloped land more arable.

 Historic Interest

Continue upstream along Crying Creek before turning away at 1.3 miles to shortly pass through an unnamed gap. A little trail leads right from the gap to the lonesome grave of Sally Sutton. Dip to a small stream before rising to reach Bear Neck Gap at 1.7 miles. ►2 The mountain slope sharpens considerably. Vines drape among the trees of a cove hardwood forest. Winter views of Three Top Mountain and Round Mountain open to the north.

Waterfall

At 2.2 miles, a spur leaves right toward Hen Wallow Falls. ►3 A profusion of rocks lies at the base of the 60-foot falls. It slides in a thin veil over a

TRAIL 23 Maddron Bald Loop Elevation Profile

stone face, before splattering into the boulder jumble. Cross Lower Falling Branch by culvert above the falls. The trail switchbacks, curves around a dry hollow, and ascends the valley of Lower Falling Branch. Reach an upper crossing of Lower Falling Branch just below a wide set of cascades. Cross it a third and last time. Notice the abundance of white quartz rocks in the streambed here.

Split a gap in Gabes Mountain at 3.3 miles. Work into the Greenbrier Creek valley, where the big trees form a forest primeval. Old-growth silverbells, buckeyes, and tulip trees shade the path. Step over small Gabes Creek. Begin winding in and out of small coves where the giants have taken their place, growing undisturbed through the American centuries.

Old–growth

East Tennessee *opens from the view down the Indian Camp Creek valley.*

⚠ Backcountry Camping

🔃 Stream

🏠 Historic Interest

Drift into Sugar Cove backcountry campsite, #34, at 4.9 miles, your first night's destination. ▶4 Multiple sites are strung along the creek. Beyond the camp, Gabes Mountain Trail climbs around Buckeye Lead, passing through a gap in a quarter mile. Big trees stand sentinel along the track. From here, the path mostly descends toward Cole Creek, which you cross twice in succession at 5.9 miles.

Drift back into settled, more level country to reach a trail intersection at 6.6 miles. ▶5 Turn left on the Maddron Bald Trail. The path slices between boulders and narrows, slipping over Maddron Creek and Jones Branch, which flow beneath the Civilian Conservation Corps–built trail. The path then passes through a small gap and shifts to the

Spruce trees rise *from the heath on Maddron Bald.*

Indian Camp Creek streamshed. Drop to the valley floor, passing rock walls and other pioneer evidence beside the trail.

Reach an old auto turnaround at mile 7.6. The path narrows yet again as it leaves the turnaround and the former civilized world. Big trees immediately tower overheard. Come to Indian Camp Creek at 8.0 miles and a long footbridge. Ascend steeply away from the creek, passing a seeping rock face that flows over the trail. The path heads toward Dunn Creek before reaching a trail junction at 8.3 miles. ▶6 Stay right with the Albright Grove Loop Trail as it circles through old-growth woods and returns to Maddron Bald Trail.

Meet the Maddron Bald Trail at 9.0 miles. ▶7 Turn right to meet Indian Camp Creek at a potentially tough crossing just above its confluence Otter Creek. Keep climbing, now along Otter Creek. Soon cross Copperhead Branch, then shortly cross Indian Camp Creek again. These crossings can be troublesome in high water.

The path curves around a relatively level cove, rife with buckeye trees, after crossing a small, unnamed feeder branch. The path curves back, looking for another creek to cross. And it soon meets Indian Camp Creek for the last time at 9.9 miles. A scenic, tiered cascade descends above the trail passage. Next, the graded trail crosses Copperhead Branch for the final time.

After leaving Copperhead Branch the path rises to the point of a ridge and a heath bald at 10.5 miles. ▶8 Look for a side trail leading left to an overlook at a rocky point. You are 4,215 feet high. Look far into East Tennessee below. To your right, Maddron Bald forms a rampart. Behind you, Old Black and the crest of the Smokies make their impressive heights known. Otter Creek, rippling down the valley below, forms the background music for the vista.

🌲 **Old-growth**

🌲 **Old-growth**

The CCC had a camp at Otter Creek in the 1930s while working on area trails.

🏞 **Waterfall**

🔭 **Great Views**

The Maddron Bald Trail leaves the vista and angles toward Otter Creek on a steep slope, working around rock outcrops. Reach Otter Creek backcountry campsite, #29, at 11.3 miles. ►9 This rationed campsite, your second night's destination, has a few flats stretched along the stream.

⚠ Backcountry Camping

The path rises to meet Maddron Bald, then becomes canopied in laurel. Make a hard right turn and continue climbing. Wind-flagged spruce trees rise from the brushy bald at 11.9 miles. ►10 Sand myrtle grows low, and spur trails head off to rock lookouts. Briefly descend, then make the last push for Snake Den Ridge Trail. Spruce trees lord over the forest.

Great Views

Meet Snake Den Ridge Trail at 12.8 miles. ►11 You are at the high point of the loop, over 5,300 feet. Continue in spruce and yellow birch amid open brush with limited vistas. Ahead, Snake Den Trail rewards hikers with views of Cosby Knob, Low Gap, and Mount Cammerer as you curve through the low-growing heath balds. Reach a notable view at 14.2 miles. ►12

Great Views

The path doesn't stay on the ridgecrest for long, as it angles back into deep green woods then switchbacks again and again, too many times to count, eventually reaching another heath bald and repeating the pattern. Pass another great view at 14.9 miles. Turn into the Inadu Creek watershed, crossing the stream at 15.6 miles. ►13 Continue down the wildflower-rich vale.

Come to an old auto turnaround. Left of the turnaround, a short path leads to a cement square, laid for forgotten reasons, and a view of Rock Creek. Cross Rock Creek by bridge at 16.5 miles. Enter the formerly settled lands of Cosby. Pass a cemetery at 16.8 miles.

⌂ Historic Interest

Reach a trail junction at 17.1 miles. ►14 Here, a horse path leaves right to meet the Low Gap Trail. Stay left on an old road, reaching Cosby

Campground near campsite, #B51, at 17.3 miles. ▶15 From here, work your way through the campground downhill to the hiker parking area. The campground walk is not included in the final trail mileage because there are numerous routes.

🚶	MILESTONES

▶1	0.0	Gabes Mountain Trailhead
▶2	1.7	Bear Neck Gap
▶3	2.2	Spur trail to Hen Wallow Falls
▶4	4.9	Campsite #34
▶5	6.6	Left on Maddron Bald Trail
▶6	8.3	Right on Albright Grove Loop Trail
▶7	9.0	Rejoin Maddron Bald Trail
▶8	10.5	View from Heath Bald
▶9	11.3	Campsite #29
▶10	11.9	Maddron Bald
▶11	12.8	Left on Snake Den Ridge Trail
▶12	14.2	View from heath bald
▶13	15.6	Cross Inadu Creek
▶14	17.1	Stay left toward Cosby Campground
▶15	17.3	Cosby Campground

Sutton Ridge Overlook

This hike to Sutton Ridge Overlook is ideal for families that want to get off the beaten path. The Lower Mount Cammerer Trail initially passes through former pioneer lands, long since forested, to reach a brook trout stream, then climbs a bit to reach Sutton Ridge. A spur trail leads to a great view of the surrounding area.

Best Time

This hike works any time of year. Each season has rewards, from wildflowers in spring, to better views of homesites in winter. The trail can be a little busier during the warm season, when Cosby Campground is open.

Finding the Trail

From Gatlinburg, take US 321 east until it comes to a T-intersection with TN 32. Follow TN 32 a little more than a mile, turning right into the signed Cosby section of the park. After 1.9 miles up Cosby Road, watch for a road splitting left to the picnic area, then the hiker parking area. Turn left here and immediately park. The Low Gap Trail starts on the upper end of the parking area.

Trail Description

Leave the Cosby hiker parking area on the Low Gap Trail. ▶1 Be apprised you can also hike the half-mile Cosby Nature Trail on your return trip. It is marked with signs at the intersection simply stating NATURE TRAIL. That path wanders through formerly settled

TRAIL USE
Dayhiking,
    Child Friendly
LENGTH
3.6 miles, 2 hours
VERTICAL FEET
+400/-400
DIFFICULTY
– 1 **2** 3 4 5 +
TRAIL TYPE
Out & Back

FACILITIES
Stream
Ridgeline
Autumn Colors
Wildflowers
Great Views
Historic Interest
Photo Opportunity

FACILITIES
(SEASONAL)
Water
Restrooms
Picnic tables
Campground

Wildflowers

In 2006, after
successful restoration
in many park streams,
brook trout streams
were reopened.

 Historic Interest

Autumn Colors

 Stream

country along Cosby Creek, which flows to your left. Cruise through a forest of maple and buckeye. Some of the hemlocks along the trail are being preserved. Pass a trail leading right toward a park employee house and the Cosby campground amphitheater (near which you can purchase a handout for the nature trail).

At 0.2 mile, keep forward as the Cosby Nature Trail forks left. Look for crumbled bits of pavement on this old road. Pass over small streams on footbridges. At 0.3 mile, the other end of the Cosby Nature Trail enters from the left. The Low Gap Trail continues forward to reach a trail junction in a flat at 0.4 mile. ▶2

Follow the Low Gap Trail just a few more steps to the Lower Mount Cammerer Trail. Keep straight, now on the wide Lower Mount Cammerer Trail, as the narrow Low Gap Trail forks right. Begin to look for evidence of settlers, such as rock walls and level areas. Tulip trees, which like to invade former fields, rise arrow straight overhead. At 0.8 mile, a short spur leads to a rocked-in spring.

At 1.3 miles, dip to Toms Creek. ▶3 This brook trout stream was once closed to fishing, as were many brook trout habitats. Brook trout are the only native Smokies trout and normally are relegated to higher elevation streams, due to heavy stocking

TRAIL 24 Sutton Ridge Overlook Elevation Profile

in the past of rainbow and brown trout. But Toms Creek, at 2,500 feet, still sports brookies.

After spanning Toms Creek on a footbridge, begin the short ascent to the nose of Sutton Ridge, which is reached at 1.7 miles. ►4 The Lower Mount Cammerer Trail continues around the ridge. There is a horse-hitching post here. The slender overlook path is lined with galax and mountain laurel. Pines grow overhead on the dry exposed ridgetop.

 Ridgeline

The path climbs then turns sharply left and switchbacks to cleared Sutton Ridge Overlook, ►5 one of the few backcountry overlooks that are kept clear. To your left and dead ahead is the upper Cosby Valley. Gabes Mountain is the prominent mountain to your left. Gilliland Ridge is to your right. Civilization lies north beyond the park boundaries.

 Great Views

On your return trip, consider taking the Cosby Nature Trail.

MILESTONES

►1	0.0	At the Cosby Hiker Parking Area, take Low Gap Trail
►2	0.4	Join Lower Mount Cammerer Trail
►3	1.3	Bridge over Toms Creek
►4	1.7	Spur to Sutton Ridge Overlook
►5	1.8	Sutton Ridge Overlook

Mount Cammerer via Low Gap

TRAIL 25

To Gatlinburg

Campsite #35

lookout tower

Rich Butt Mountain

Gabes Mountain Trail

start & finish

P

Cosby Campground

Lower Mount Cammerer Trail

Panther Branch

Toms Creek

GREAT SMOKY MOUNTAINS NATIONAL PARK

TENNESSEE
NORTH CAROLINA

Low Gap Trail

Rocky Face Mountain

Cosby Creek

Rough Montain

Low Gap

Low Gap Trail

Camel Hump Branch

Dry Branch

N

Big Branch
Riding Fork
Cosby Park Road
Cosby Creek
Sutton Ridge
Toms Creek

Robinson Creek
Gilliland Fork
Gilliland Ridge

Rowdy Creek
Groundhog Creek
McFalls Branch

0   0.2   0.4   0.6 miles
0 0.2 0.4 0.6 kilometers

Mount Cammerer via Low Gap

Revel at great views from a historic restored lookout tower. Leave Cosby Campground, and head up Cosby Creek valley through gorgeous woodland to the state line. Meet the Appalachian Trail at Low Gap. Cruise the state line to emerge at an outcrop and tower where the world falls away.

Best Time

Hikers find their way to Mount Cammerer year-round. Fall through spring offer the most far-reaching views. Summer afternoons can be stormy.

Finding the Trail

From Gatlinburg, take US 321 east until it comes to a T-intersection with TN 32. Follow TN 32 a little more than a mile, turning right into the signed Cosby section of the park. After 1.9 miles up Cosby Road, watch for a road splitting left to the picnic area, then the hiker parking area. Turn left here and immediately park. The Low Gap Trail starts on the upper end of the parking area.

Trail Description

Called "White Rock" by Tennesseans and "Sharp Top" by Carolinians before the park's inception, this mountaintop rock outcrop was named in perpetuity for Arno B. Cammerer, former director of the National Park Service. No matter the name, this sentinel has incredible panoramas from its place on the Smokies crest. A historic wood and stone fire

TRAIL USE
Dayhiking
LENGTH
11.2 miles, 5–7 hours
VERTICAL FEET
+2,780/-2,780
DIFFICULTY
– 1 2 3 4 **5** +
TRAIL TYPE
Out & Back

FEATURES
Stream
Ridgeline
Summit
Autumn Colors
Wildflowers
Great Views
Geologic Interest
Historic Interest
Photo Opportunity

SEASONAL FACILITIES
Water
Restrooms
Picnic tables
Campground

tower, long in disuse, has been restored by a group known as Friends of the Smokies. This restoration makes Mount Cammerer an even more desirable destination.

The trail's beginning, within the greater realm of Cosby Campground, can be a bit confusing, with numerous trail junctions in the first half mile. But exercise a little persistence and soon you are ascending the gorgeous valley of Cosby Creek, where tall trees shade mossy boulders and Cosby Creek forms a watery attraction alongside which wildflowers grow in spring. It is a steady climb to Low Gap, but the trail is in good shape. From there, the AT has its ups, but the hardest part to Cammerer is over.

Leave the hiker parking area ▶1 and drop to an old path of crumbling asphalt. Cosby Creek is downhill to your left. Soon pass the campground amphitheater. A cold piped spring is on trail left just before the amphitheater. The now lovely woodland around you was once farmland. The path soon splits as the Cosby Nature Trail meanders through the woods to the left. Stay with the signs indicating Low Gap, passing over two creeks via footbridges. The second creek is Cosby Creek. Reach the upper part of the Cosby Nature Trail. This time stay right. The Low Gap Trail soon reaches an open area and the Lower Mount Cammerer Trail at 0.4 mile. ▶2

 Stream

TRAIL 25 Mount Cammerer via Low Gap Elevation Profile

Leave the trail junction and continue climbing toward Low Gap. This area was also once farmland, but is now rich in wildflowers. Pass a water-monitoring station on Cosby Creek just before reaching a trail junction at 0.8 mile. Here, a connector trail leads 0.4 mile back to Cosby Campground and 0.6 mile to Snake Den Ridge Trail. This connector allows hikers and equestrians to avoid the campground if they are going to Snake Den Ridge.

 Wildflowers

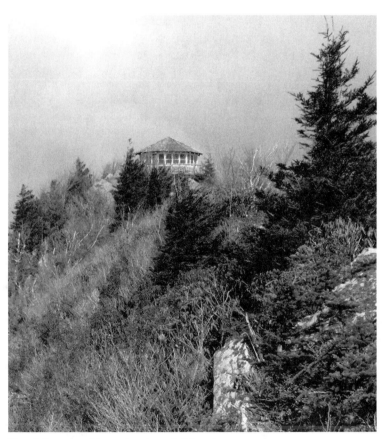

Mount Cammerer Tower *rises above wind-flagged spruce trees.*

Friends of the
Smokies, a private
support group working
in concert with the
park, restored the
lookout tower.

Stay with the Low Gap Trail, continuing the steady but not too steep uptick toward the Smokies crest, now in tall woodland. You are walking the old maintenance road to the Mount Cammerer fire tower. The wide track allows you to look around more rather than watch your every step. Tulip trees, maple, preserved hemlock, and black birch form a green cathedral overhead. Moss and ferns grow on the boulder-strewn ground, which becomes a wildflower garden in spring. Come back alongside Cosby Creek, where pretty cascades form white ribbons dropping between mossy boulders.

At mile 1.3, the trail makes the first of several switchbacks, leaving the dark creekside world behind. The ascent steepens as the trail works the slopes of Rocky Face Mountain to your left. Cross a tributary at 1.8 miles. ▶3 Keep rising. Step over now-tiny Cosby Creek again at mile 2.4. ▶4

Geologic Interest

The Low Gap Trail works around rock outcrops. The last stretch is a straight shot to make Low Gap and the Appalachian Trail at mile 2.9. ▶5 The elevation here is 4,242 feet. At Low Gap, turn left, northbound on the AT, and resume your ascent. A mile of steady climbing leads through northern hardwoods of cherry and yellow birch, along with scattered spruce. The Appalachian Trail levels out near Sunup Knob at mile 4.0. ▶6 Winter views of the heath balds along lower Mount Cammerer open. Then trail is as level as they come in the Smokies, rising slightly near the junction with the Mount Cammerer Trail at mile 5.0. ▶7

▲ **Ridgeline**

Follow the Mount Cammerer Trail along the state line ridge into mountain laurel. The AT drops toward Davenport Gap. After a slight dip, reach the outcrop and tower at mile 5.6. ▶8 You don't need to get in the tower to enjoy the vistas from the jutting rocks—you can see in every direction. However, the inside of the octagonal structure provides refuge from winds.

Summit

Great Views

The rock cut of I-40 is visible to your east, and the road follows the Pigeon River. Mount Sterling and its metal fire tower rises to your south. In the foreground to your north is the appropriately named Stone Mountain. Beyond Stone Mountain, Tennessee stretches until the horizon's end. Maybe a place this spectacular deserves three names.

👤	MILESTONES	
▶1	0.0	At the Cosby Hiker Parking Area, take Low Gap Trail
▶2	0.4	Lower Mount Cammerer Trail leaves left
▶3	1.8	Step over tributary
▶4	2.4	Cross uppermost Cosby Creek
▶5	2.9	Low Gap
▶6	4.0	Sunup Knob
▶7	5.0	Mount Cammerer Trail
▶8	5.6	Mount Cammerer

Twentymile and Fontana Lake Area

Twentymile and Fontana Lake Area

The Twentymile and Fontana Lake area is the least accessible and least visited area of the Smokies. The dearth of nearby towns, boater-only accesses, and long, winding drives combine to keep the crowds down. Located in the most northwesterly section of the North Carolina Smokies, this area includes three major drainages that flow south from the state line ridge: Twentymile, Hazel, and Eagle Creeks. Fontana Lake forms the south boundary. The Appalachian Trail traverses most of the state line crest. Elevations range from higher than 5,000 feet along the state line down to 1,300 feet at Twentymile Ranger Station. Fontana Lake stands 1,710 feet at full pool. Eagle Creek and Hazel Creek flow into Fontana Lake, while Twentymile Creek feeds Cheoah Lake. Hazel Creek is laden with history. A little more than a century ago, a timber town, Proctor, harbored more than 1,000 residents who worked lumbering operations. Today, the forest has recovered, and Hazel Creek is now known as the Smokies' most storied trout fishery. Rough, remote Eagle Creek requires many fords to travel its watershed. Both of these creeks are accessed primarily by boat on Fontana Lake, including a fee shuttle operating out of Fontana Marina. Landlocked hikers can access this area from the north side of Fontana Dam, Twentymile Ranger Station, and over the mountain crest from Tennessee.

All the watersheds are noteworthy not only for fishing but simply for national park–level magnificence. Twentymile Creek and its major tributary, Moore Spring Branch, exhibit deep, above-average-size pools divided by seemingly ceaseless cascades. Eagle Creek exudes a back-of-beyond wild aura and a slender hiker-only path that epitomizes backcountry. Hazel Creek is one of the largest streams in the park. Its tributary network avails water lovers more opportunities to explore aquatic scenery and the verdant woodlands that surround them, combined with human history.

The high country is too low for spruce-fir. It is instead cloaked in northern hardwoods in most places. An exception is the most famous

Fontana Lake *as seen from Shuckstack fire tower (Trail 28)*

Southern Appalachian mountain meadow of them all—Gregory Bald. This grassy clearing, punctuated with blueberry bushes and wild azaleas, reveals pronounced views, berries in season, and the most colorful display of flame azaleas on the planet. This is one of two balds being preserved by the park, the other being Andrews Bald, near Clingmans Dome. Yet even better views can be had atop Shuckstack Mountain, where one of two historic park fire towers is preserved. This destination on the Appalachian Trail presents a 360-degree panorama of the Smokies crest, Fontana Lake, and the Nantahala National Forest to the south.

All park camping in this area is backcountry only. Car campers can overnight at Cable Cove or Tsali Campgrounds in the Nantahala National Forest on Fontana Lake's south shore. Paddlers and boaters can camp at boat-only backcountry campsites on the lake and also lakeside hiker-accessible sites. Area trails are generally lesser used, except for the AT.

When boating to a trailhead, plan ahead, whether you are using your own boat or a shuttle. Fontana Marina and Cable Cove are the two best boat-launching options for exploring the Fontana Smokies. Also, be apprised that Fontana Lake generally is at full pool from late May through early September. Lower lake levels make accessing the lake trailheads a little tougher, and may require scrambling over open, potentially muddy lakebed.

Permits

Permits are *not* required for dayhiking. Backpackers, however, must get a backcountry permit to stay at one of the 23 designated backcountry campsites located in this area. Most require a simple self-registration; however, others require a reservation, which you can make by calling the backcountry permit office at (865) 436-1231. Pick up and fill out backcountry permits at Twentymile Ranger Station, Fontana Marina, and Fontana Dam Visitor Center, run by Tennessee Valley Authority.

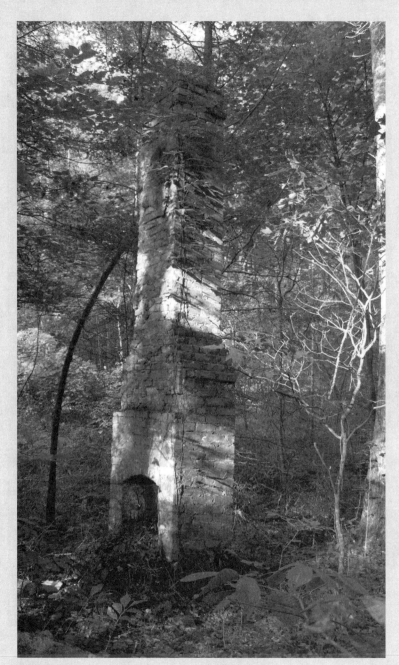

Sunlight filters *onto a lonely chimney from a time forgotten.*

Twentymile and Fontana Lake Area

Mill Creek

Parson Branch Road

Mount Squires

High Point ▲

Eagle Creek

Gregory Little Bald ▲

TENNESSEE

NORTH CAROLINA

GREAT SMOKY MOUNTAINS NATIONAL PARK

▲ Parsons Bald

Big Swag ▲

Twentymile Creek

Round Mountain Knob ▲

The Pinnacle ▲

Sheep Knob ▲

Little Shuckstack ▲

To **321** and Townsend, TN

26 27 28

Eagle Creek

Big Butte ▲

30 31

Matt Mountain ▲

Hazel Creek

28

Fontana Dam ▲

29

Little Tennessee River

Fontana Lake

Round Mountain ▲

To Bryson City

High Top ▲

28

Yellow Creek

Perry Knob ▲

Yellow Creek Road

Yellow Creek

129

N

| 0 | 1 | 2 | 3 miles |
| 0 | 1 | 2 | 3 kilometers |

TRAIL FEATURES TABLE

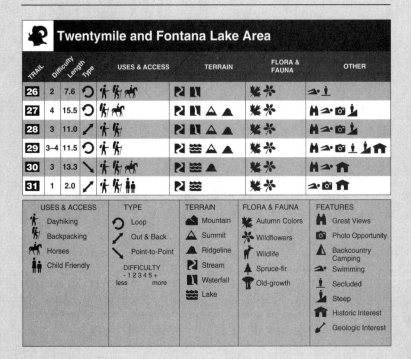

Twentymile and Fontana Lake Area

TRAIL	Difficulty	Length	Type	USES & ACCESS	TERRAIN	FLORA & FAUNA	OTHER
26	2	7.6	Loop	Dayhiking, Backpacking, Horses	Stream, Waterfall	Autumn Colors, Wildflowers	Swimming, Secluded
27	4	15.5	Loop	Backpacking, Horses	Stream, Waterfall, Summit, Ridgeline	Autumn Colors, Wildflowers	Great Views, Swimming, Photo Opportunity, Steep
28	3	11.0	Out & Back	Dayhiking, Backpacking	Stream, Waterfall, Summit, Ridgeline	Autumn Colors, Wildflowers	Great Views, Swimming, Photo Opportunity, Steep
29	3–4	11.5	Loop	Dayhiking, Backpacking	Stream, Lake, Summit, Ridgeline	Autumn Colors, Wildflowers	Great Views, Swimming, Photo Opportunity, Secluded, Steep, Historic Interest
30	3	13.3	Point-to-Point	Dayhiking, Backpacking, Horses	Stream, Lake, Ridgeline	Autumn Colors, Wildflowers	Great Views, Swimming, Historic Interest
31	1	2.0	Out & Back	Dayhiking, Backpacking, Child Friendly	Stream, Lake	Autumn Colors, Wildflowers	Swimming, Photo Opportunity, Historic Interest

USES & ACCESS	TYPE	TERRAIN	FLORA & FAUNA	FEATURES
Dayhiking	Loop	Mountain	Autumn Colors	Great Views
Backpacking	Out & Back	Summit	Wildflowers	Photo Opportunity
Horses	Point-to-Point	Ridgeline	Wildlife	Backcountry Camping
Child Friendly	DIFFICULTY	Stream	Spruce-fir	Swimming
	- 1 2 3 4 5 +	Waterfall	Old-growth	Secluded
	less more	Lake		Steep
				Historic Interest
				Geologic Interest

Maps

For the Twentymile and Fontana Lake area, here are the USGS 7.5-minute (1:24,000-scale) topographic quadrangles that you will need, listed in the order that you will need them as you hike along your route.

Trail 26: Tapoco, Fontana Dam
Trail 27: Tapoco, Fontana Dam, Cades Cove, Calderwood
Trail 28: Tapoco, Fontana Dam
Trail 29: Fontana Dam
Trail 30: Tuskegee, Fontana Dam
Trail 31: Tuskegee

Twentymile and Fontana Lake Area

Twentymile Loop 191
Leave a quiet trailhead to circle past Twentymile Cascades. Bisect dry ridges to reach Moore Spring Branch watershed. Numerous footlog bridge stream crossings present panoramas of deep pools and frothier cascades.

Gregory Bald Loop 197
Ascend Twentymile Creek, passing Twentymile Cascades and along dark pools before leaving the stream. Make Gregory Bald, with its views and world-renowned wild azalea displays. Camp below the bald at Sheep Pen Gap. Pass over what remains of Parson Bald, and return via Moore Spring Branch, with its plentiful cascades.

Shuckstack from Twentymile Ranger Station 205
This is one of the better climb-it-because-it-is-there hikes. Leave Twentymile Ranger Station, travel along pool-and-drop Twentymile Creek, and pass Twentymile Cascades. Climb from the valley onto a dry ridgeline, meeting the Appalachian Trail. A final ascent leads to a restored metal fire tower with a stupendous 360-degree view.

Lost Cove Loop 211
This loop makes for a rewarding but long dayhike or good backpack. Travel the history-sprinkled Lakeshore Trail with many pre-park relics. Enjoy views of Fontana Lake. Climb along secluded Lost Cove Creek to the Appalachian Trail. Reach astonishing vistas from atop Shuckstack fire tower. Trace the AT down to the trailhead and Fontana Lake.

TRAIL 29

Dayhiking, Backpacking

11.5 miles, Loop

Difficulty: 1 2 **3** 4 5

Fontana Lake Hike 217
Regularly done as a dayhike, this trip can be an excellent backpack for water lovers and backpack beginners. Take a boat shuttle to Hazel Creek and piney creekside camp. Follow Lakeshore Trail past old homesites to Eagle Creek and a lakeside camp. Pass more pioneer history as the Lakeshore Trail delivers you to Fontana Dam.

TRAIL 30

Dayhiking, Horses, Backpacking

13.3 miles, Point-to-Point

Difficulty: 1 2 **3** 4 5

Ruins of Proctor 225
Take a boat shuttle on scenic Fontana Lake to Hazel Creek. Make an easy stroll to a backcountry camp, once the lumber town of Proctor. Explore the former townsite, heading up Hazel Creek to reach the relics of a mill, now covered in forest. Discover other area sites, including the Calhoun House.

TRAIL 31

Dayhiking, Backpacking, Child Friendly

2.0 miles, Out & Back

Difficulty: **1** 2 3 4 5

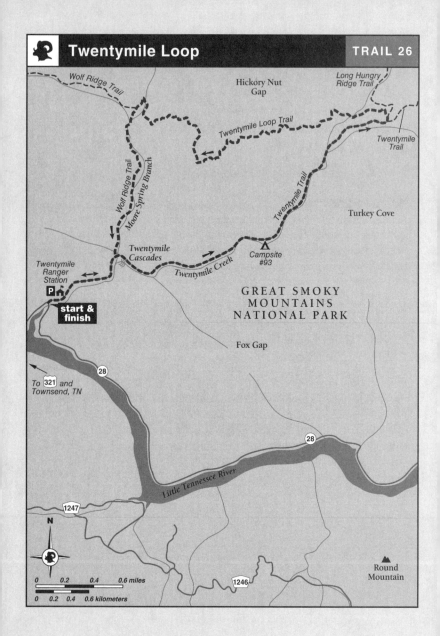

Twentymile Loop

TRAIL 26

Wolf Ridge Trail

Hickory Nut Gap

Long Hungry Ridge Trail

Twentymile Loop Trail

Twentymile Trail

Wolf Ridge Trail

Moore Spring Branch

Twentymile Trail

Turkey Cove

Twentymile Cascades

Campsite #93

Twentymile Ranger Station

P

start & finish

Twentymile Creek

GREAT SMOKY MOUNTAINS NATIONAL PARK

Fox Gap

28

To 321 and Townsend, TN

28

Little Tennessee River

1247

N

Round Mountain

1246

0   0.2   0.4   0.6 miles

0   0.2   0.4   0.6 kilometers

Twentymile Loop

Leave a quiet trailhead to circle past Twentymile Cascades. Bisect dry ridges to reach Moore Spring Branch watershed. Numerous footlog bridge stream crossings present panoramas of deep pools and frothier cascades.

Best Time

Late winter and spring offer the most water to enjoy Twentymile Cascades and all the other unnamed falls on Twentymile Creek and Moore Spring Branch. The watersheds are also rich wildflower areas.

Finding the Trail

From Townsend, Tennessee, take US 321 north to the Foothills Parkway. Follow Foothills Parkway west to US 129. Follow US 129 south into North Carolina to reach NC 28. Follow NC 28 south for 2.6 miles to Twentymile Ranger Station, on your left.

From US 19/74 near Bryson City, take US 19 south to NC 28. Veer right and join NC 28 south 30 miles to Twentymile Ranger Station, which will be on your right, after passing Fontana Dam.

Trail Description

This streamside loop hike never gets too far from the sound of falling water, a key ingredient that makes the Smokies what they are. First, walk along Twentymile Creek, with its big pools that far outsize the amount of water it carries to Cheoah Lake. Stay

TRAIL USE
Dayhiking, Horses,
   Backpacking
LENGTH
7.6 miles, 3½–4½ hours
VERTICAL FEET
+1,300/-1,300
DIFFICULTY
– 1 **2** 3 4 5 +
TRAIL TYPE
Loop

FEATURES
Stream
Waterfalls
Autumn Colors
Wildflowers
Swimming
Secluded

FACILITIES
Picnic table
Camping

with the Twentymile Trail, shortly reaching the tiered Twentymile Cascades, an accessible waterfall that is fun to play around. Continue up the stream, bridging Twentymile Creek numerous times, getting looks into the fast-dropping stream as it dashes white through a green cathedral. Make a trail junction at now-grown Proctor Field Gap. Veer left on the hiker-only Twentymile Loop Trail, bridging Twentymile Creek one last time. Rise into silent wooded Long Hungry Ridge. Moore Spring Branch, a fine trout stream, serenades your downgrade. A short back-track leads you to the trailhead.

Start your loop on the Twentymile Trail on a wide roadlike path. ▶1 Twentymile Creek stair-steps south for Cheoah Lake. A forest of beech, black birch, and rhododendron rises from the ferny forest floor. Your hillside vantage allows views into the deep pools of Twentymile Creek, bordered by mossy rocks. The stream carries a higher amount of sediment relative to other Smoky Mountain streams and thus has a brownish tint. The sediment also causes the stream to cloud up after thunderstorms. **Stream** However, it doesn't affect the fishery. Feisty rainbow trout can be found in every pool. A skilled angler will have a ball battling these colorful fish. At 0.5 mile, bridge Moore Spring Branch just before it meets Twentymile Creek. Reach a trail junction. ▶2

TRAIL 26 Twentymile Loop Elevation Profile

Turn right, staying with Twentymile Trail, as the Wolf Ridge Trail, your return route, leaves left. Make a short quick climb then reach the spur trail to Twentymile Cascades. ▶3 From the main path you can already gain a wide perspective of the cascades as they drop 40 or so feet over a distance of 30 yards, making multiple falls and rock slides into multiple pools divided by multiple ledges. The largest descent is the last one, as the creek pours over

Waterfall

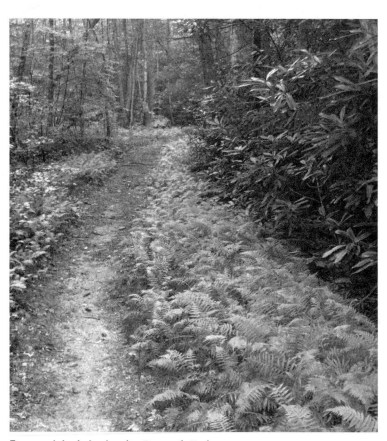

Ferns and rhododendron *line Twentymile Trail.*

a sloped rock slab. Ample dunking pools beckon. Smooth gray sunning rocks avail a spot to dry.

Resume your ascent along Twentymile Creek, which continues splashing over big boulders into shadowy pools, backed against a rising wall of rhododendron. Scan for big boulders scattered in the forest. Bridge the stream at 1.5 miles, and again at 1.7 miles to reach Twentymile Creek backcountry campsite, #93. ►4 It is located in a flat on the curve of the stream. The main trail bridges Twentymile Creek again at the upper end of the campsite at 1.8 miles.

Cross a stream flowing out of Turkey Cove at 2.2 miles. Rise deeper into the mountains. Span Twentymile Creek at 2.5 miles, just below a boulder-strewn cascade. Watch for a big gravel bar and pool before bisecting the stream again at 2.6 miles. Here, the path turns away from the creek into piney woods to reach Proctor Field Gap and a trail junction at 3.2 miles. ►5 The forest has overtaken the field from which it drew a name. Here, the hiker-only Twentymile Loop Trail leaves left, while the Long Hungry Ridge Trail keeps straight for Campsite #92. The Twentymile Trail leaves right for the Appalachian Trail.

Take the narrow Twentymile Loop Trail as it drifts downhill to bridge an unnamed streamlet. Next, cross Twentymile Creek on a footlog. Here, the force of the stream pounds into a mossy stone bluff then slows as a pool before pushing over boulders. The path weaves up Long Hungry Ridge in dry forest of white pine, oak, and hickory. The secluded woodland is an ideal place for contemplative solitude, to absorb the essence of the Southern Appalachians. Split a gap on Long Hungry Ridge at 4.5 miles. Continue in upland forest. Bisect a second gap at 4.9 miles. ►6 Views open across the valley of Wolf Ridge.

Descend to reach Moore Spring Branch at 5.8 miles in a rocky glen, where a five-foot curtain drops

▲ Backcountry Camping

Ť Secluded

into a deep pool. Turn down Moore Spring Branch and join the Wolf Ridge Trail at 5.9 miles. ▶7 Keep downstream, bridging Moore Spring Branch on foot-logs at 6.0, 6.3, 6.6, 6.7, and 6.8 miles. They are fun to cross because they also give you enhanced vistas into the water. Deep pools, rock slides, and white frothy cascades cloaked in greenery characterize this superlatively scenic Smoky Mountain stream. Pass by a rare-for-the-Smokies dry rock overhang just before your loop ends at 7.1 miles. ▶8 It is but a half-mile backtrack to the trailhead. ▶9

 Stream

🚶	**MILESTONES**	
▶1	0.0	Twentymile Trailhead
▶2	0.5	Right with Twentymile Trail
▶3	0.6	Twentymile Cascades
▶4	1.8	Campsite #93
▶5	3.2	Twentymile Loop Trail
▶6	4.9	Gap in Long Hungry Ridge
▶7	5.9	Join Wolf Ridge Trail
▶8	7.1	Right on Twentymile Trail
▶9	7.6	Twentymile Trailhead

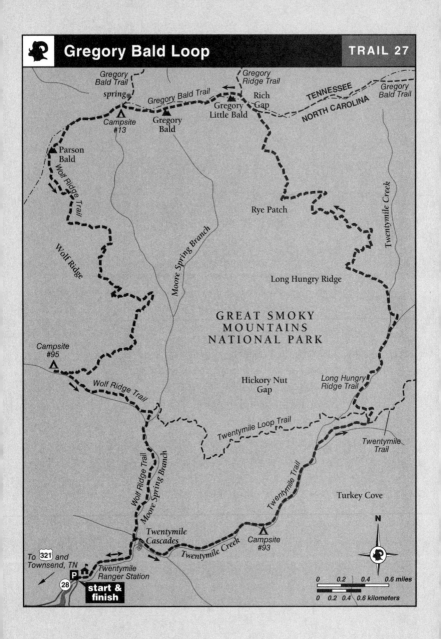

Gregory Bald Loop

TRAIL 27

Gregory Bald Trail
Gregory Bald Trail
spring
Gregory Ridge Trail
Rich Gap
Gregory Little Bald
TENNESSEE
NORTH CAROLINA
Gregory Bald Trail
Campsite #13
Gregory Bald
Parson Bald
Wolf Ridge Trail
Wolf Ridge
Rye Patch
Moore Spring Branch
Twentymile Creek
Long Hungry Ridge
GREAT SMOKY MOUNTAINS NATIONAL PARK
Campsite #95
Wolf Ridge Trail
Hickory Nut Gap
Long Hungry Ridge Trail
Twentymile Loop Trail
Twentymile Trail
Wolf Ridge Trail
Moore Spring Branch
Twentymile Trail
Turkey Cove
N
Twentymile Cascades
Twentymile Creek
Campsite #93
To 321 and Townsend, TN
P
28
Twentymile Ranger Station
start & finish

0   0.2   0.4   0.6 miles
0   0.2 0.4   0.6 kilometers

Gregory Bald Loop

Ascend Twentymile Creek, passing Twentymile Cascades and along dark pools before leaving the stream. Make Gregory Bald, with its views and world-renowned wild azalea displays. Camp below the bald at Sheep Pen Gap. Pass over what remains of Parson Bald, and return via Moore Spring Branch, with its plentiful cascades.

Best Time

June is the time to be on Gregory Bald to see the flame azaleas. Early August is better for picking blueberries. Views are best in fall after the first cool fronts sweep through. Winter and spring bring good views also, but the weather up top can be iffy.

Finding the Trail

From Townsend, Tennessee, take US 321 north to the Foothills Parkway. Follow Foothills Parkway west to US 129. Follow US 129 south into North Carolina to reach NC 28. Follow NC 28 south for 2.6 miles to Twentymile Ranger Station, on your left.

Alternate directions: From US 19/74 near Bryson City take US 19 south to NC 28. Veer right and join NC 28 south 30 miles to Twentymile Ranger Station, which will be on your right, 7.7 miles after passing the turn to the Fontana Dam Marina and Visitor Center.

Trail Description

This hike combines the best the high and low country have to offer. Four backcountry campsites allow

TRAIL USE
Backpacking, Horses
LENGTH
15.5 miles, 9–11 hours
VERTICAL FEET
+3,570/-3,570
DIFFICULTY
– 1 2 3 **4** 5 +
TRAIL TYPE
Loop

FEATURES
Summit
Ridgeline
Stream
Waterfall
Autumn Colors
Wildflowers
Great Views
Swimming
Steep
Photo Opportunity

FACILITIES
Picnic table

197

backpackers to vary the mileage and length of their trips. Those in topnotch mountain hiking shape can do it as a strenuous dayhike. The Twentymile Trail leads through a magnificent stream valley past Twentymile Cascades then Twentymile Creek campsite and on to Upper Flats campsite, both available for overnight stays. A little more creekside hiking leads to an arduous climb, topping out on Long Hungry Ridge at Rye Patch. From there, ramble high ridges to make Gregory Bald, the Southern Appalachians most famed highland meadow, with its staggering views and flower displays. High country camping is an option at Sheep Pen Gap, a grassy glade shaded with yellow spruce, below Gregory Bald.

Your return route passes nearly overgrown Parson Bald. Leave the state line via the steep Wolf Ridge Trail, negotiating never-ending switchbacks. Pass isolated Dalton Branch campsite, another overnight alternative, before crisscrossing Moore Spring Branch, with its deep pools and stair-step falls. Be apprised that Sheep Pen Gap campsite, #13, the busiest site on this circuit, requires a phone-in reservation.

Twentymile Trail ▶1 rises above Twentymile Creek, flowing below in alternating pools and rapids.

 Stream

Rich woods pocked with big boulders shade the

TRAIL 27 Gregory Bald Loop Elevation Profile

track. At 0.5 mile, Moore Spring Branch flows in from your left. ▶2 Bridge the creek just before beginning the loop portion of the hike. Stay right with the Twentymile Trail, as the Wolf Ridge Trail, your return route, leaves left. Shortly come to Twentymile Cascades. ▶3 A series of ledges divides pools, culminating in a rock slide at the base of the cascade.

 Waterfall

Continue hiking up Twentymile Creek, admiring more cascades and trout-filled pools, half-hidden behind rhododendron and black birch. Bridge the stream at 1.5, 1.7, and 1.8 miles. Twentymile Creek backcountry campsite, #93, is located in a flat just before the bridge at 1.8 miles. ▶4 Bridge Twentymile Creek twice more at 2.5 miles

Wildflowers

Backcountry Camping

Gregory Bald *presents a feast of mountains from its grassy crest.*

and 2.6 miles. The path temporarily leaves Twentymile Creek, ascending through pines to make Proctor Field Gap and a trail junction at 3.2 miles. ►5

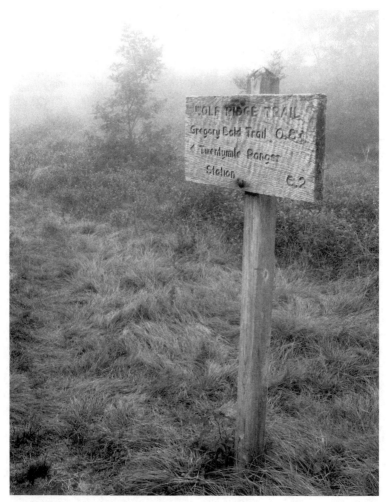

Parson Bald, *once a grassy meadow, is all but grown over.*

Stay straight and pick up the Long Hungry Ridge Trail, dipping to step over Proctor Branch. Swing around the point of a ridge, then dip alongside Twentymile Creek again. At 4.3 miles, reach Upper Flats backcountry campsite, #92, elevation 2,520. ▶6 Upper Flats has several good tent sites from which to choose, at its perch between Twentymile Creek and Greer Branch. Large rocks emerge from the ground, forming natural seats at the camps.

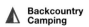

Backcountry Camping

Beyond Upper Flats immediately rock-hop Twentymile Creek, then step over Rye Patch Branch. The once moderate grade steepens as the trail crosses Rye Patch Branch a final time at 4.9 miles, your last easy water. Ascend a dry ridge slope amid oaks. Partial views open to the southeast. Make sharp switchbacks at 5.5, 6.2, and 6.4 miles. Level off at Rye Patch, 4,400 feet, at 6.7 miles. This once open area is mostly overgrown, but remains an ideal resting spot after you have climbed to the crest of Long Hungry Ridge.

Steep

Ridgeline

The balance of the Long Hungry Ridge Trail is easy, ending in Rich Gap and the Tennessee state line at 7.6 miles. ▶7 Turn left on the Gregory Bald Trail, walking the state line on what was the Appalachian Trail before Fontana Dam was built. Northern hardwoods such as buckeye, cherry, and beech rise over a grassy floor.

The park service maintains grassy, brushy Gregory Bald, dotted with wind-sculpted trees at its present 15-acre size.

Reach another trail junction at 7.7 miles. ▶8 If you are thirsty, take the unmarked left route 0.3 mile to tasty Moore Spring, the site of an old Appalachian Trail shelter. Continue straight on the Gregory Bald Trail and climb 0.6 mile to the grassy meadow of Gregory Bald at 8.3 miles. ▶9 A nearly 360-degree view opens. Cades Cove lies below to the north. Flame azaleas bloom in June and blueberries follow after that. The bald is large and has many elements, so allow time to explore it all.

Great Views

Reenter woods on the western end of the bald, descending to the Wolf Ridge Trail junction and

Backcountry Camping

Sheep Pen Gap backcountry campsite, #13, elevation 4,560, at 8.8 miles. ►10 The grassy glade of open level woodland is one of the Smokies' finer backcountry locales. However, it is very heavily used and requires reservations. You can get water by walking 200 yards down the Gregory Bald Trail to a spring. Sunset from atop Gregory Bald is a Smoky Mountains sight to see.

Continue the loop, heading southwest on the Wolf Ridge Trail through level woodland, making a slight uptick before making Parson Bald at 9.6 miles. ►11 The park service is not maintaining this bald, unlike Gregory Bald. It has grown up with trees and blueberry and azalea bushes, limiting views but proffering colorful beauty. All too soon you have passed through the bald remnants.

 Wildflowers

 Steep

Leave the state line into North Carolina, beginning an irregular but steep descent down Wolf Ridge, punctuated with frequent switchbacks amid oaks. Watch for white quartz pebbles on the trail. Come within earshot of Moore Spring Branch at 11.8 miles, only to turn away from the stream on a sharp switchback.

 Backcountry Camping

Dip toward Dalton Branch, meeting the quarter-mile side trail leading to Dalton Branch backcountry campsite, #95, at 13.1 miles. ►12 Veer left and pick up an old road leading to the Twentymile Loop trail junction at 13.9 miles. Bridge Moore Spring Branch five times on fun footlogs, admiring the pools and falls of the watercourse, to arrive at the Twentymile Trail junction at 15.0 miles. ►13 Retrace the Twentymile Trail 0.5 mile to the trailhead, ►14 completing your loop.

MILESTONES

►1	0.0	Twentymile Trailhead
►2	0.5	Right with Twentymile Trail
►3	0.6	Twentymile Cascades
►4	1.8	Campsite #93
►5	3.2	Straight on Long Hungry Ridge Trail
►6	4.3	Campsite #92
►7	7.6	Left on Gregory Bald Trail
►8	7.7	Pass the spur to Moore Spring
►9	8.3	Gregory Bald
►10	8.8	Campsite #13, left on Wolf Ridge Trail
►11	9.6	Parson Bald
►12	13.1	Spur to Campsite #95
►13	15.0	Twentymile Trail
►14	15.5	Twentymile Trailhead

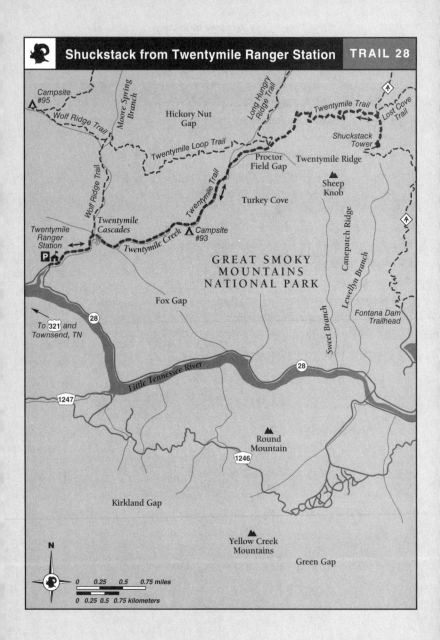

Campsite #95

Moore Spring Branch

Wolf Ridge Trail

Hickory Nut Gap

Long Hungry Ridge Trail

Twentymile Trail

Lost Cove Trail

Shuckstack Tower

Twentymile Loop Trail

Proctor Field Gap

Twentymile Ridge

Wolf Ridge Trail

Twentymile Trail

Sheep Knob

Twentymile Cascades

Turkey Cove

Twentymile Ranger Station

Twentymile Creek

Campsite #93

Canepatch Ridge

GREAT SMOKY MOUNTAINS NATIONAL PARK

Fox Gap

Lewellyn Branch

To 321 and Townsend, TN

28

Sweet Branch

Fontana Dam Trailhead

Little Tennessee River

28

1247

1246

Round Mountain

Kirkland Gap

N

Yellow Creek Mountains

Green Gap

0   0.25   0.5   0.75 miles

0 0.25 0.5 0.75 kilometers

Shuckstack from Twentymile Ranger Station

This is one of the better climb-it-because-it-is-there hikes. Leave Twentymile Ranger Station, travel along pool-and-drop Twentymile Creek, and pass Twentymile Cascades. Climb from the valley onto a dry ridgeline, meeting the Appalachian Trail. A final ascent leads to a restored metal fire tower with a stupendous 360-degree view.

TRAIL USE
Dayhiking, Backpacking
LENGTH
11.0 miles, 6–8 hours
VERTICAL FEET
+2,660/-2,660
DIFFICULTY
– 1 2 **3** 4 5 +
TRAIL TYPE
Out & Back

FEATURES
Stream
Waterfall
Ridgeline
Summit
Autumn Colors
Wildflowers
Great Views
Swimming
Steep
Photo Opportunity

FACILITIES
Picnic table

Best Time

The clear skies of fall and winter avail the farthest-reaching views from Shuckstack Tower. In winter the cascades of Twentymile Creek may be frozen, adding a wintry treat to the trek. Views in summer can be hazy.

Finding the Trail

From Townsend, Tennessee, take US 321 north to the Foothills Parkway. Follow Foothills Parkway west to US 129. Follow US 129 south into North Carolina to reach NC 28. Follow NC 28 south for 2.6 miles to Twentymile Ranger Station, on your left.

Alternate directions: From US 19/74 near Bryson City take US 19 south to NC 28. Veer right and join NC 28 south 30 miles to Twentymile Ranger Station, which will be on your right, after passing Fontana Dam.

Trail Description

A sure, steady, but not too steep path leads from the lowlands of Twentymile Ranger Station to the metal fire tower atop Shuckstack Mountain, where an above-the-treetops vista awaits from one of two preserved fire towers within the park boundaries. The flora changes with the elevation, adding vegetational variety to the trek. The hike isn't as daunting as the mileage may indicate. Anybody in decent shape can—with ample rest breaks—make this hike. It is uphill the whole way, but downhill all the way back!

 Stream

The wide Twentymile Trail ►1 ascends astride Twentymile Creek, which falls in a pool-drop-pool fashion. The deep pools of Twentymile Creek harbor lively rainbow trout. At 0.5 mile, bridge Moore Spring Branch above its confluence with Twentymile Creek. ►2 Beyond the bridge, stay right with the Twentymile Trail, as the Wolf Ridge Trail heads left. A brief uptick leads to the spur trail to Twentymile Cascades. ►3 Look down as the cataract descends 40 feet in stair-step fashion over wide stone ledges. In summer you could get wet in a pool then dry off on a sunny rock. The water will feel especially good after a sweaty climb in the Southern humidity.

Waterfall

The trail continues mimicking the curves and gradient of Twentymile Creek. Big boulders stand among the hardwoods, while the northeast-facing side of the valley is cloaked in thickets of rhododendron. Doghobble finds its trailside place. This

Wildflowers

TRAIL 28 Shuckstack from Twentymile Ranger Station Elevation Profile low, arching shrub grows only in the Southern Appalachians. In late spring doghobble produces clusters of small, bell-shaped flowers that droop from its arms. The waist-high thickets prove quite an impediment for most creatures, including people and dogs. In pioneer days, hunted bears would crash through such thickets using their powerful bodies, losing the dogs that were in pursuit of them, giving the plant its name, doghobble.

Bridge the stream at 1.5 miles, then at 1.8 miles to reach the Twentymile Creek backcountry campsite, #93. ▶4 The overnighting locale is located in a flat bordered by the stream on one side and a rising hill on the other. The Twentymile Trail

Backcountry Camping

Looking toward the main crest *of the Smokies from Shuckstack fire tower*

bridges Twentymile Creek again at the upper end of the campsite, then rises well above the stream. Bridge a creeklet flowing out of Turkey Cove at 2.2 miles, and continue penetrating farther into the park. Bridge Twentymile Creek at 2.5 miles, just below a boulder-strewn cascade. Watch for a big gravel bar and pool before bridging the stream again at 2.6 miles. Here, the path turns away from the creek, rising in piney woods to reach Proctor Field Gap and a trail junction at 3.2 miles. ▶5 Resting logs are scattered at the intersection.

Bear right at the trail junction, staying on the Twentymile Trail. The path now parallels Proctor Branch, flowing off to your left, while small rills flow under the now narrower trail. The woods still reflect a streamside habitat. Cross your last trickle at 3.9 miles. The going is higher and drier as you make your way into xeric woods of oak, mountain laurel, pines, sourwood, sassafras, and blueberry bushes.

 Stream

Sassafras trees are easy to identify. Their leaves have three basic shapes: oval, three-lobed, and mitten-shaped. Mature sassafras trees have a reddish-brown, deeply furrowed bark. They are known for their aromatic scent. Scratch the bark from a twig and the sweet smell is unmistakable. American natives used sassafras for medicinal purposes. Pioneers made tea by boiling the roots, and some people still do today. Birds eat the berries. The wood of sassafras shrinks when dried and is used for fence posts and hand tools. Sassafras roots were one of the first exports from the American colonies to Europe.

___

Shuckstack resembles the piles of discarded cornstalks (stacks of corn shucks) gathered by farmers for winter cattle feed.

___

Though you are climbing, this is about as good as climbing gets, with the steady grade and good footing. Dark galax leaves line the path. Twentymile Ridge rises to your right. Keep looking upward along that ridge for the slender tower of Shuckstack. In winter the views are clear, but even when the leaves are on you can spot it. The final ascent to the Appalachian Trail is completed in a series of switch-

 Autumn Colors

backs to arrive at Sassafras Gap at 5.1 miles. ▶6 This four-way trail junction is another spot where tower seekers take a break.

Turn right, southbound, on the more heavily trodden Appalachian Trail. Meander a minute before climbing from Sassafras Gap and skirting the north slope of Shuckstack. Emergent rocks rise from the steep mountainside. Reach the spur to Shuckstack at 5.4 miles. ▶7 The acute left turn rises up the craggy knob 0.1 mile to the top of Shuckstack and a fire tower, elevation 4,020 feet. ▶8 The chimney from the tower watcher's cabin stands quiet. The concrete cistern reflects a time when, during the spring and fall fire seasons, these towers would be manned.

 Summit

Atop the tower, views extend in every direction. The main crest of the Smokies and state line is northeast. Fontana Lake covers the flooded valley of the Little Tennessee River to the southeast. The rampart of Gregory Bald stands to the northwest. Your route up the Twentymile Creek valley lies to the southwest. Waves of mountains extend southward into the Nantahala National Forest. From this vantage point, the surrounding Southern Appalachians look especially rugged. Soak up the views before backtracking to the trailhead.

 Great Views

 Photo Opportunity

🚶	MILESTONES	
▶1	0.0	Twentymile Trailhead
▶2	0.5	Right with Twentymile Trail
▶3	0.6	Twentymile Cascades
▶4	1.8	Campsite #93
▶5	3.2	Proctor Field Gap
▶6	5.1	At Sassafras Gap, turn right, southbound, on the AT
▶7	5.4	Left on spur to Shuckstack
▶8	5.5	Fire tower with 360-degree view

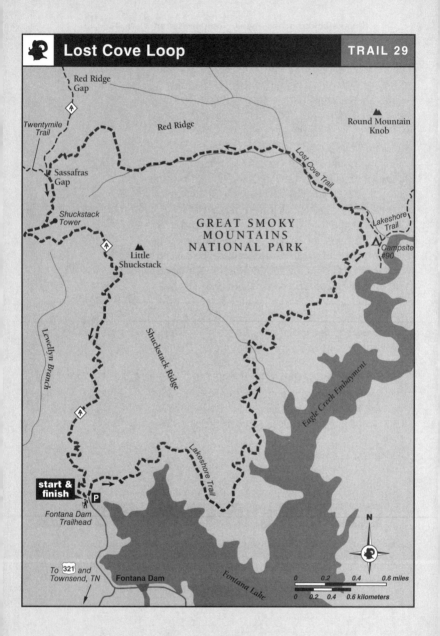

Lost Cove Loop

TRAIL 29

Red Ridge Gap

Twentymile Trail

Red Ridge

Round Mountain Knob

Lost Cove Trail

Sassafras Gap

Shuckstack Tower

Lakeshore Trail

GREAT SMOKY MOUNTAINS NATIONAL PARK

Campsite #90

Little Shuckstack

Llewellyn Branch

Shuckstack Ridge

Eagle Creek Embayment

Lakeshore Trail

start & finish

P

Fontana Dam Trailhead

To 321 and Townsend, TN

Fontana Dam

Fontana Lake

N

| 0 | 0.2 | 0.4 | 0.6 miles |

| 0 | 0.2 | 0.4 | 0.6 kilometers |

Lost Cove Loop

This loop makes for a rewarding but long dayhike or good backpack. Travel the history-sprinkled Lakeshore Trail with many pre-park relics. Enjoy views of Fontana Lake. Climb along secluded Lost Cove Creek to the Appalachian Trail. Reach astonishing vistas from atop Shuckstack fire tower. Trace the AT down to the trailhead and Fontana Lake.

Best Time

Winter offers clear skies for gaining views atop Shuckstack fire tower and also allows more looks into pioneer relics along the Lakeshore Trail. In spring, the part of the loop along the Appalachian Trail can be busy with thru-hikers. Fall has clear skies and solitude.

Finding the Trail

From Townsend, Tennessee, take US 321 north to the Foothills Parkway. Follow the Foothills Parkway to US 129. Turn south on US 129 into North Carolina. Turn left on NC 28 south, passing Fontana Village. Go 1.5 miles past the Fontana Village entrance, and turn left at the sign to Fontana Dam. Follow the signs to Fontana Dam, crossing the dam, then stay right just beyond the dam to dead end at the trailhead, 2.2 miles from NC 28.

Alternate directions: From Bryson City, North Carolina, take US 19/74 south to NC 28. Follow NC 28 south to the intersection with NC 143. Zero your trip odometer here and continue on NC 28 south. It is 9.9 miles on NC 28 to the right turn to Fontana Dam. Follow the signs to Fontana Dam, crossing the

TRAIL USE
Dayhiking, Backpacking
LENGTH
11.5 miles,
6½–8½ hours
VERTICAL FEET
+3,100/-3,100
DIFFICULTY
– 1 2 **3** 4 5 +
TRAIL TYPE
Loop

FEATURES
Ridgeline
Summit
Stream
Lake
Autumn Colors
Wildflowers
Great Views
Swimming
Steep
Photo Opportunity
Secluded
Historic Interest

FACILITIES
Picnic tables
Restrooms
Water

dam, then stay right just beyond the dam to dead end at the trailhead, 2.2 miles from NC 28.

Trail Description

This loop can be a full day's hike or easily stretched into an overnight backpack. It is also a great Smokies sampler hike. It presents pre-park history, lake views, mountain streams, old homesites, and ridge running and is capped off with a great view from a fire tower accessed via the Appalachian Trail. You start at the Fontana Dam Trailhead ▶1 following a former highway reverted to wilderness because of the dam's construction. Roller-coaster over rib ridges divided by streams flowing into Fontana Lake.

Reach Lost Cove Creek, with backcountry camping. You have the option of walking downstream to meet the Eagle Creek arm of Fontana Lake before traveling up secluded Lost Cove. A steep final ascent brings you to Sassafras Gap and the Appalachian Trail. One last uptick reaches Shuckstack fire tower and a panorama that rewards every uphill step you took. Views stretch as far as the clarity of the sky allows. From the top of the tower it's all downhill. Pass a natural vista from a rock face. The AT switchbacks down a dry ridge, leveling off at occasional gaps, before returning to the lowlands near Fontana Dam.

TRAIL 29 Lost Cove Loop Elevation Profile

Take the Shuttle or Camp near the Lake

OPTIONS

Bypass the 5.1-mile Lakeshore Trail segment and get a boat shuttle from Fontana Marina, landing at Lost Cove backcountry campsite, #90. Then take the Lakeshore Trail up to meet Lost Cove Trail and aim for Shuckstack.

Depending on the lake levels, the shuttle will drop you off near Lost Cove backcountry campsite, #90. Here you can explore Lost Cove Creek, Fontana Lake, and the Eagle Creek while overnighting on the lake.

Pick up the Lakeshore Trail as it follows the wide bed of old North Carolina 288. This area wasn't originally slated to be part of the Smoky Mountains National Park. It was added only after Fontana Lake was to be built to furnish power for the Alcoa aluminum plant in Maryville, Tennessee, for the World War II effort. The land around the dam and Fontana Lake was condemned and purchased by the federal government. The land on the north side of the impoundment was then deeded over to the park, making the boundary at Fontana Lake's edge. This was all hastefully done before World War II. That is why this area has more "modern" relics and evidence such as this wide highway grade and even roadside jalopies.

Oaks dominate the forest, along with plentiful tulip trees regenerating even atop the roadbed. Creek bottoms are clothed in rhododendron and birch. Step over Payne Branch at 0.8 mile, ▶2 then ascend to surmount a gap. Descend along a trickling tributary. Watch for some big holly trees here. Pass the ruins of an old car near a fast disappearing farm **Historic Interest** clearing; walnut trees are reclaiming the field.

Rejoin the old auto highway at 1.5 miles. ▶3 Ahead more rusty hulks of vehicles lie abandoned along the old road. Views of the Eagle Creek embayment open to your right through the pines. Leave **Great Views** the road for the final time at 2.4 miles. ►4 Stay left here, traveling straight up a rhododendron-shaded branch, crossing the stream, then climbing to a gap. This pattern will soon repeat itself many times over.

Bisect streams at 3.0, 3.1, and 3.5 miles, the last being Birchfield Branch. ►5 More stream and ridge undulations occur. The lake seems but an illusion at this point. Eventually Lost Cove Creek rushes audibly below. A few switchbacks deliver you to Lost Cove Creek Trail at 5.1 miles. ►6

This loop turns left up the Lost Cove Trail. The dark hollow is tight here, and Lost Cove Creek plummets over mossy boulders into pools. Rock-hop the creek three times in the next 0.2 mile. The valley widens and you enter Lost Cove, where several homes once were. Watch for a partial stone chimney to the right of the trail at 5.6 miles. More crossings lie ahead—if the water is high your feet will get wet. Under normal flows the stream can be easily rock-hopped. You probably won't realize it, but you rock-hop Cold Springs Branch, the major tributary of Lost Cove Creek, before reaching Upper Lost Cove backcountry campsite, #91, at 5.8 miles. ►7 The site is sloped but offers seclusion in a vale of spring wildflower profusion.

The slender footpath steepens beyond the campsite. Stream crossings ease up, until you are stepping over more rock than water. The path turns away from what is left of Lost Cove Creek at 6.9 miles and ascends steeply. A few switchbacks ease the climb. Huff and puff your way into Sassafras Gap at 7.8 miles. ►8 The small gap beckons a rest.

Turn left, southbound on the Appalachian Trail. It shows much more use than Lost Cove Trail. A brief level stretch is followed by an assault on the boulder-strewn north flank of Shuckstack. Reach the spur trail to the fire tower at 8.2 miles. Stay left and switchback up the rocky summit to reach the fire tower and old lookout cabin site at 8.3 miles. ►9

🔁 Stream

🏠 Historic Interest

⚠️ Backcountry Camping

👤 Steep

👤 Summit

The chimney and water cistern mark the site of what was a job offering a lot of solitude. Climb the metal tower. Undulating panoramas open in all directions. You can see Fontana Lake, the Lost Cove Creek valley, the main chain of the Smokies, Twentymile Creek valley, and the wall of Gregory Bald in the background. Looks like that firewatcher job came with a few perks!

Return to the narrow hiker-only Appalachian Trail, and continue southbound. Make a sharp-switchback then pass an open stone face offering natural southern vistas. Drop to a gap betwixt Shuckstack and Little Shuckstack at 9.2 miles. ▶10 Continue the downgrade, briefly entering a hollow to step over a trickling stream at 10.0 miles. ▶11 Occasional westerly views of Fontana Lake open. The switchbacks continue under the hickories and oaks. Emerge at the Fontana Dam Trailhead at 11.5 miles, ▶12 completing the loop.

 Great Views

Rangers, staffing these fire towers, lived in them full time during the spring and fall fire seasons.

🚶 MILESTONES

▶1	0.0	Fontana Dam Trailhead
▶2	0.8	Payne Branch
▶3	1.5	Old highway
▶4	2.4	Leave old highway
▶5	3.5	Birchfield Branch
▶6	5.1	Left on Lost Cove Trail
▶7	5.8	Campsite #91
▶8	7.8	Left on Appalachian Trail
▶9	8.3	Shuckstack fire tower
▶10	9.2	Gap between Shuckstack and Little Shuckstack
▶11	10.0	Trickling stream
▶12	11.5	Fontana Dam Trailhead

Fontana Lake Hike

TRAIL 30

Hazel Creek Trail

Lakeshore Trail

Big Ridge

Calhoun House

Campsite #86

Trail 26

boat shuttle drop-off

Campsite #88

Lakeshore Trail

Big Butte

Hazel Creek

Matt Mountain

GREAT SMOKY MOUNTAINS NATIONAL PARK

Eagle Creek Trail

Campsite #90

Eagle Creek

Fontana Lake

Lakeshore Trail

Lost Cove Trail

Little Shuckstack

Shuckstack Ridge

Cable Cove Boat Ramp

28

trail shelter

Fontana Marina

P

start & finish

Fontana Dam

Fontana Dam Trailhead

28

28

To 321 and Townsend, TN

N

1.5 miles

1.5 kilometers

0   0.5   1

0   0.5   1

Fontana Lake Hike

Regularly done as a dayhike, this trip can be an excellent backpack for water lovers and backpack beginners. Take a boat shuttle to Hazel Creek and piney creekside camp. Follow Lakeshore Trail past old homesites to Eagle Creek and a lakeside camp. Pass more pioneer history as the Lakeshore Trail delivers you to Fontana Dam.

Best Time

Fontana Lake is at full pool during summer and is its most scenic. Swimming also is good then. Spring offers cooler temperatures and wildflowers. Winter is a poor choice because of annual lake drawdowns.

Finding the Trail

From Townsend, Tennessee, take US 321 north to the Foothills Parkway. Follow the Foothills Parkway to US 129. Turn south on US 129 into North Carolina. Turn left on NC 28 south, passing Fontana Village. Go 1.5 miles past the Fontana Village entrance, and turn left at the sign to Fontana Dam. Next, turn right at the sign to Fontana Village Marina a short distance away.

Alternate directions: From Bryson City, North Carolina, take US 19/74 south to NC 28. Follow NC 28 south to the intersection with NC 143. Zero your trip odometer here and continue on NC 28 south. It is 9.9 miles on NC 28 to the right turn to Fontana Dam. Shortly turn right at the sign to Fontana Village Marina. Follow the road over the dam, veering right after the dam to reach the Fontana Dam Trailhead 2.2 miles from NC 28.

TRAIL USE
Backpacking,
    Dayhiking, Horses

LENGTH
13.3 miles, 7–9 hours

VERTICAL FEET
+1,860/-1,840

DIFFICULTY
– 1 2 **3** 4 5 +

TRAIL TYPE
Point-to-Point

FEATURES
Lake
Ridgeline
Stream
Autumn Colors
Wildflowers
Great Views
Swimming
Historic Interest

FACILITIES
Picnic tables
Restrooms
Water
Camping

217

Trail Description

If you like a combination of mountains, streams, and lakes, this hike is for you and any younger or inexperienced backpackers you may wish to bring along. It is a doable as a dayhike, but you best get started early. Be apprised this trip takes planning; you must arrange a boat shuttle to the trailhead. Contact Fontana Marina at (828) 498-2211, extension 277, to arrange for a one-way fee shuttle; you will hike back to the marina. Also, both recommended backcountry campsites on this route require phone-in reservations with the park service. The boat shuttle ▶1 takes you on a pleasure ride from Fontana Marina to Hazel Creek, where you see wave upon wave of mountains from a watery grandstand.

Your drop-off point is where Hazel Creek flows into Fontana Lake. Backpackers can walk a mere half mile to a pine-shaded campsite on the banks of Hazel Creek. Talk about an easy first day! Use your free time to explore the old townsite of Proctor, fish Hazel Creek, swim in the lake, or relax at camp.

From there, the hike leads west up historic Possum Hollow where settler evidence abounds. Surmount Pinnacle Ridge to reach Eagle Creek, a tumultuous mountain rill. Ahead, another campsite

TRAIL 30 Fontana Lake Hike Elevation Profile

lies at the confluence of Eagle Creek, Lost Cove Creek, and Fontana Lake. Simultaneously enjoy tumbling streams and a mountain-rimmed lake.

The final part of the hike bisects rib ridges extending from Shuckstack Mountain divided by tumbling watersheds, all mixed in with still more homesites, and even a few old jalopies left from pre-park days. Intersect the Appalachian Trail, and walk over Fontana Dam to Fontana Marina, completing a water and woods loop.

The boat shuttle drops you off at the mouth of Hazel Creek. Soak in mountain vistas on the ride, for the lake trip is part of this overall experience. The **Lake**

Waves of mountains *rise from Fontana Lake.*

Hazel Creek Trail, shaded by black birch, sycamore, and ferns aplenty, takes you to Proctor backcountry campsite, #86, at 0.5 mile. ▶2 White pines carpet the camp with needles as cool Hazel Creek rushes by. Soon reach a wide bridge and trail junction.

⚠ **Backcountry Camping**

Cross the bridge and stay left, taking the Lakeshore Trail toward the Calhoun House, owned

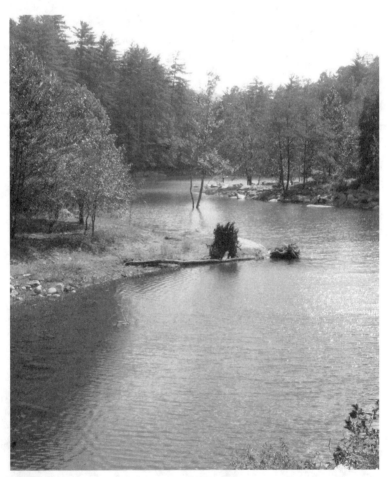

Fontana Lake *snakes into the mountains near Campsite #90.*

and used by the park. Pass the house, climbing a bluff only to descend back to Hazel Creek. Turn into Possum Hollow at 1.2 miles. ▶3 Remnants of the old community of Proctor, including relic fields, train axles, chimneys, and foundations, are very evident along this valley of Sheehan Branch.

 Historic Interest

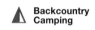 **Wildflowers**

Continue up an old wagon road, passing spurs to pioneer cemeteries. The gently ascending trail narrows. Pass the spur trail to Campsite #88 at 2.0 miles. ▶4 This small, less than ideal camp is on a slope. An intact brick chimney stands just ahead. Continue along an ever-diminishing watercourse to reach a gap in Pinnacle Ridge at 3.1 miles.

 Backcountry Camping

From here, the Lakeshore Trail follows a graded park-created path, rather than a historic pioneer track. Descend through hickory, oak, pine, and mountain laurel woods, occasionally coasting into lonely hardwood coves. Watch for quartz-encrusted boulders beside the trail at 3.9 miles. Entertain sporadic lake views. The cry of Eagle Creek accompanies a few final switchbacks, and you reach the Eagle Creek Trail at 5.1 miles. ▶5

 Stream

Turn left to descend along boulder-sprinkled Eagle Creek, still on the Lakeshore Trail. Cross an iron trestle bridge and soon Fontana Lake comes into view. Pass over Lost Cove Creek on a footlog to arrive at strategically located and busy Lost Cove backcountry campsite, #90, at 5.5 miles. ▶6 This oak- and hickory-shaded camp offers fishing and swimming in both Fontana Lake and the mountain streams nearby. A network of user-created trails makes finding the continuance of the Lakeshore Trail a challenge. As you look out on the lake from the campsite, the Lakeshore Trail is uphill and to your right, entering the Lost Cove Creek valley.

 Backcountry Camping

Travel up the cool rhododendron-dominated valley. Turbulent Lost Cove Creek crashes below. Reach the Lost Cove Trail junction at 6.0 miles. ▶7 Stay left with the Lakeshore Trail, climbing to the first of innumerable gaps dividing drainages into Fontana Lake. This portion of the Lakeshore Trail has many old roads and trails leading off it, so make sure you stay on the right path. Fontana Lake is on your left the whole way.

The trail follows a familiar pattern: up and around a point of a ridge, and down into a creek-filled hollow, up the side of a ridge and over the point, and down again into a hollow. Step over Birchfield Branch at 7.6 miles. ►8 Intersect a former road, Old NC 28, at 8.7 miles. ►9 It still has some junker cars from the 1930s nearby. Homesites and other evidence of human habitation are all around this section of trail. Enjoy views of Fontana Lake from piney points. Leave the old road at 9.6 miles, ►10 heading right to pass through a fast disappearing farm clearing. Bisect a gap then return to the old roadbed. Emerge at the Fontana Dam Trailhead at 11.1 miles. ►11

Road walk and reach the north side of Fontana Dam at 11.7 miles. ►12 Cross Fontana Dam, appreciating the immensity of the project and the views of Fontana Lake. Follow the Appalachian Trail to the left away from Fontana Dam Road and reenter woodland. Pass a trail shelter known as the Fontana "Hilton," because it was considered fancy when first erected. After running a low ridgeline through thick woods, the AT crosses a road leading to the marina. The marina is a short distance downhill to your left. Turn left on the road and complete your loop at 13.4 miles. ►13

 Autumn Colors

 Historic Interest

Fontana Dam is the highest dam east of the Mississippi River.

Great Views

🚶 MILESTONES

▶1	0.0	Fontana Marina (boat shuttle departure point)
▶2	0.5	Campsite #86
▶3	1.2	Possum Hollow
▶4	2.0	Campsite #88
▶5	5.1	Eagle Creek Trail
▶6	5.5	Campsite #90
▶7	6.0	Lost Cove Trail
▶8	7.6	Birchfield Branch
▶9	8.7	Meet old NC 28
▶10	9.6	Leave old NC 28
▶11	11.1	Pass Fontana Dam Trailhead
▶12	11.7	Fontana Dam
▶13	13.4	Fontana Marina

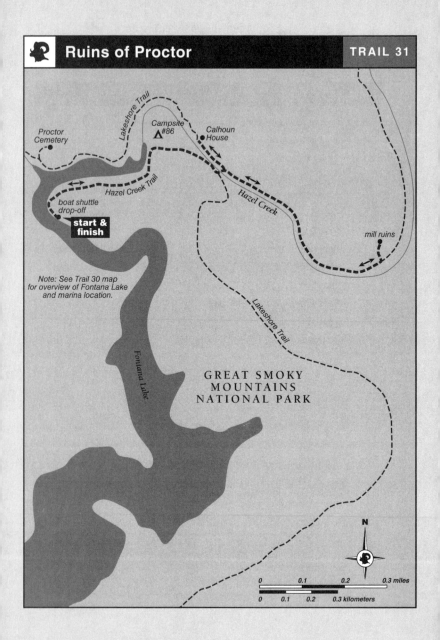

Proctor
Cemetery

Lakeshore Trail

Campsite
#86

Calhoun
House

boat shuttle
drop-off

Hazel Creek Trail

**start &
finish**

Hazel Creek

mill ruins

Note: See Trail 30 map
for overview of Fontana Lake
and marina location.

Lakeshore Trail

Fontana Lake

GREAT SMOKY
MOUNTAINS
NATIONAL PARK

N

| 0 | 0.1 | 0.2 | 0.3 miles |

| 0 | 0.1 | 0.2 | 0.3 kilometers |

Ruins of Proctor

Take a boat shuttle on scenic Fontana Lake to Hazel Creek. Make an easy stroll to a backcountry camp, once the lumber town of Proctor. Explore the former townsite, heading up Hazel Creek to reach the relics of a mill, now covered in forest. Discover other area sites, including the Calhoun House.

Best Time

Late spring and summer are the best times to enjoy the boat ride on Fontana Lake. Warm weather also favors exploring the waters of Hazel Creek. The easy trail is enjoyable any time of year.

Finding the Trail

From Townsend, Tennessee, take US 321 north to the Foothills Parkway. Follow the Foothills Parkway to US 129. Turn south on US 129 into North Carolina. Turn left on NC 28 south, passing Fontana Village. Go 1.5 miles past the Fontana Village entrance, and turn left at the sign to Fontana Dam. Turn right at the sign to Fontana Village Marina a short distance away.

From Bryson City, North Carolina, take US 19/74 south to NC 28. Follow NC 28 south to the intersection with NC 143. Zero your trip odometer here and continue on NC 28 south. It is 9.9 miles on NC 28 to the right turn to Fontana Dam. Shortly turn right at the sign to Fontana Village Marina.

TRAIL USE
Dayhiking, Backpacking,
  Child Friendly
LENGTH
2.0 miles, 4–6 hours,
  including boat
  shuttle
VERTICAL FEET
+70/-70
DIFFICULTY
– **1** 2 3 4 5 +
TRAIL TYPE
Out & Back

FEATURES
Lake
Stream
Autumn Colors
Wildflowers
Historic Interest
Swimming
Photo Opportunity

FACILITIES
Restrooms
Water

Trail Description

Great Smoky Mountains National Park has a few tourist towns in its shadow. The towns have T-shirt shops, restaurants, museums, games, and rides—many swirling climbing, splashing, round-and-round rides. If you want to lure your offspring to the park to feast upon the natural beauty contained within its boundaries, take them on this walk. It starts with a boat ride!

Take a boat shuttle from Fontana Marina, located far from the tourist towns, and cruise Fontana Lake. The crest of the Smokies rises on one side, while the peaks of the Nantahala National Forest flank the other. Narrow coves slice high green ridges. You will travel easterly along the impoundment, which dammed the waters of the Little Tennessee River.

The sinuous lake stretches as far as the eye can see, but you turn northeasterly up the Hazel Creek embayment. Welch Ridge and Matt Mountain peer down from above. If you can turn your head away from the mountains and look into the water, you'll notice the lake's unbelievable clarity—rocks, submerged logs, and fish are visible 20 or more feet deep. The Hazel Creek embayment narrows, twists, and turns its last mile or so, following the course of the streambed underneath. Thickly wooded

Great Views

Lake

TRAIL 31 Ruins of Proctor Elevation Profile

OPTIONS

Proctor Cemetery

Hike a half mile beyond the Calhoun House on the Lakeshore Trail to reach the spur to Proctor Cemetery. Many homesites and settler evidence are up Possum Hollow beyond the cemetery.

ridges crowd the now slender waterway. Soon the sounds of Hazel Creek rushing to meet the waters of Fontana Lake reach your ears.

It's time to jump off the boat and explore the ruins of Proctor. This boat ride and stroll through the Smoky Mountains past leaves everybody with a smile on their face and the contrived rides of the tourist towns forgotten.

This adventure requires planning. Contact Fontana Marina at (828) 498-2211, extension 277, to arrange for a drop-off and pickup shuttle. I recommend starting early to get the most for your money—the shuttle isn't cheap, but it's a unique way to enjoy the Smoky Mountains National Park. It takes around an hour to hike to the mill ruins and back to the boat drop-off. If you start early, you will have plenty of time to explore the place at your leisure, have a picnic, fish, and swim in Fontana Lake or in the chilly waters of the Baptism Pool, a deep section of Hazel Creek.

By the way, since a backcountry campsite is located a half mile from the boat drop-off, anyone interested in camping can simply carry their gear from the lake to the campsite without needing a backpack or any specialized gear. In fact, campers here bring so-called luxury items such as camp chairs and coolers. Consider bringing less physically able campers to the site to experience the Smokies backcountry. You can simply arrange your pickup for the next day—or the day after. This campsite, #86, requires a phone-in reservation.

In the 1830s Moses Proctor settled near the town that was to bear his name. Others filtered in, farmers mostly. Small-scale mining and lumber operations took place. But in 1907, the Southern Railway ran through the nearby Little Tennessee River Valley, allowing easier access to Proctor. Ritter Lumber Company bought large tracts of land in the Hazel Creek Valley, then ran a spur rail line up Hazel Creek. They established a lumber boomtown at once sleepy Proctor. The population grew to more than a thousand people, with all the services needed to feed, house, and entertain the lumbermen and their families.

By 1928, the town had peaked. An estimated 200 million board feet of lumber had been cut, processed, and shipped out on the railroad. The townspeople followed the lumber. At this time there was already talk of a national park being established here. By the mid-1940s the entire valley was left to the beasts of the Smokies. The forest has recovered nicely, though signs of the logging days are visible.

Your exact drop-off spot may vary, depending on the lake level. ▶1 Immediately join the Hazel Creek Trail, traveling a wide gravel path. A canopy of black birch, red maple, and rhododendron borders the track. The stream drains the North Carolina high country west of Clingmans Dome. Hazel Creek, a storied fishing venue, is one of the bigger watercourses in the park.

At 0.5 mile, you reach the signpost for Campsite #86, Proctor. ▶2 To your left, trails lead under the big white pines that drop their fragrant needles on the large camping flat. This was once the playground for Proctor School, where the children of the lumbermen were educated. The school stood on the hill to your right as you stand at the campsite signpost. Sometimes it's hard to imagine that civilization once held fast in these now-wooded hills. But if you

Stream

Backcountry Camping

Historic Interest

walk around, you will find artifacts large and small. Leave them for others to discover and enjoy.

Reach a trail junction and bridge at 0.6 mile. ▶3 Ahead, the Lakeshore Trail briefly follows what was Struttin' Street in the Proctor days, before leaving east for Forney Creek. Cross the bridge, then turn left on the Lakeshore Trail, heading downstream along Hazel Creek to reach the Calhoun House, built in 1923. I have seen the home locked and closed and other times open for exploration. The Park Service formerly used it in their operations, but now it is kept as a purely historic building. The huge white oaks in front of the house saw Proctor in its heyday.

Now backtrack to the bridge, this time heading up the Hazel Creek Trail. Note the old field to your left, growing up in walnut trees. Look for squared-off flat spots, old roadbeds, metal washtubs, and other imprints of Proctor. You are now circling around the huge flat upon which the lumber mill, trains, logs, boards, and attendant facilities stood. What once was a loud and noisy place has reverted back to nature but still holds its past underneath the brush and trees.

At 1.0 mile, look left for a clear trail leading into the woods away from Hazel Creek. The path travels a berm between former log ponds. Shortly reach the brick and concrete mill ruins, ▶4 along with assorted junk, even a bathtub. *As with any abandoned structures, look around but be careful.* Notice how nature is reclaiming the area, with trees growing in, around, and over the ruins.

Stream

Historic Interest

🚶	**MILESTONES**	
▶1	0.0	Boat drop-off at the mouth of Hazel Creek
▶2	0.5	Campsite #86
▶3	0.6	Bridge over Hazel Creek
▶4	1.0	Mill ruins

Deep, Forney, and Noland Creeks Area

Deep, Forney, and Noland Creeks Area

The Deep, Forney, and Noland Creeks area is comprised of three major drainages that flow from the highest point in the park, Clingmans Dome, into North Carolina near Bryson City. A variance in flora and fauna characterize the extreme elevation changes. Altitudes range from higher than 6,600 feet along the state line ridge dividing North Carolina and Tennessee down to 1,700 feet near the park entrance at Deep Creek and the full pool level of Fontana Lake. Both Forney Creek and Noland Creek flow into Fontana Lake. Deep Creek flows into the Tuckasegee River, which flows into Fontana Lake. Up high, you will encounter one of the larger swaths of Canadian-type spruce-fir forest, an ice age relic cloaking only the highest mantles of the park. The spruce-fir zone includes not only the main crest, but also the upper ridges that divide the streamsheds—Forney Ridge, Noland Divide, and Thomas Divide.

Descending in elevation, the forest types blend into northern hardwoods, cove hardwoods, and pine-oak on drier sites. Along the streams, dense temperate jungles of black birch, yellow birch, sycamore, and tulip trees rise above massive thickets of rhododendron and doghobble. The crystalline streams crash over rocks, occasionally slowing to form pools where trout furtively ply a rich subaquatic food chain.

The lower portions of these now deeply wooded valleys were once settled by pre-park pioneers, who gave their names to many of the tributaries: Bumgardner Branch, Huggins Creek, and more. In addition to being settled, parts of the area were logged, from a small-scale selective cutting operation on Deep Creek to a near-complete forest takedown using railroads on Forney Creek. The woodland has recovered well from both pioneer settlement and timber operations. Ironically, hikers use many of the old timber harvesting railroad grades for trails. Later, the Civilian Conservation Corps enhanced or otherwise created more trails, some of which unfortunately have been abandoned.

Overleaf and opposite: Verdant forests rise in the hills and hollows of the Great Smoky Mountains.

The streams and ridges attract hikers, backpackers, equestrians, anglers, tubers, and campers who overnight at Deep Creek Campground. Visitors also stay in Bryson City, adjacent to the park. The hikes described are primarily loops, including both dayhikes and overnight treks. The area's primary features—the vista at Andrews Bald, the spruce-fir forests, several waterfalls on gorgeous streams, a slice of Fontana Lake, and pioneer homesteads—can be seen here. Hikers enter the high country from Clingmans Dome Road. Hikers enter the "lowlands" near Bryson City, from the Deep Creek Campground and day-use area, as well as Lakeview Drive, also known as the Road to Nowhere.

Permits

Permits are *not* required for dayhiking. Backpackers, however, must get a backcountry permit to stay at one of the 23 designated backcountry campsites located in this area. Most require a simple self-registration; however, others require a reservation, which you can make by calling the backcountry permit office at (865) 436-1231. Pick up and fill out backcountry permits at Deep Creek Campground entrance station. If you're traveling in the high country, obtain your permit at Oconaluftee Visitor Center when coming from North Carolina, or Sugarlands Visitor Center when coming from Tennessee.

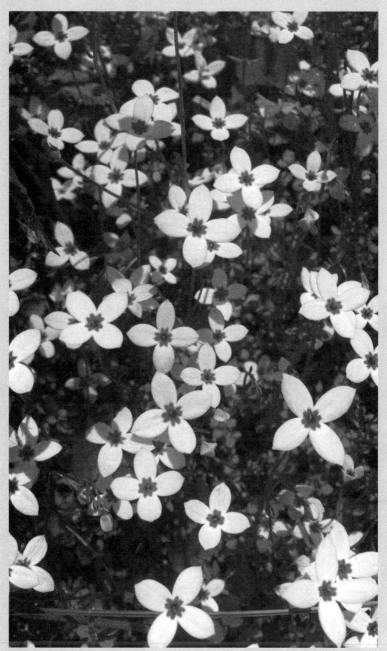

Bluets brighten *the trailside on the way to Andrews Bald (Trail 39).*

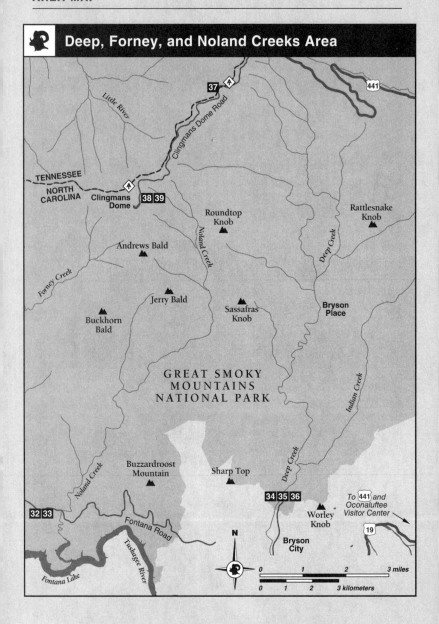

Deep, Forney, and Noland Creeks Area

Deep, Forney, and Noland Creeks Area

TRAIL	Difficulty	Length	Type	USES & ACCESS	TERRAIN	FLORA & FAUNA	OTHER
32	2	3.2	Loop	Dayhiking, Backpacking, Horses	Stream, Lake	Autumn Colors, Wildflowers	Swimming, Historic Interest, Secluded
33	2	8.8	Loop	Dayhiking, Backpacking, Horses	Stream, Lake, Summit	Autumn Colors, Wildflowers	Great Views, Swimming, Historic Interest
34	3	12.0	Loop	Dayhiking, Backpacking, Horses	Stream, Waterfall, Ridgeline	Autumn Colors, Wildflowers	Historic Interest, Secluded
35	1–2	2.4	Loop	Dayhiking, Child Friendly	Stream, Waterfall	Autumn Colors, Wildflowers	Swimming, Photo Opportunity, Historic Interest
36	5	22.5	Loop	Backpacking, Horses	Stream, Waterfall, Ridgeline	Autumn Colors, Wildflowers, Wildlife	Swimming, Historic Interest, Secluded
37	5	20.1	Loop	Backpacking, Horses	Stream, Ridgeline	Autumn Colors, Wildflowers, Spruce-fir	Great Views, Swimming, Secluded, Steep
38	5	19.4	Loop	Backpacking, Horses	Stream, Waterfall, Ridgeline	Autumn Colors, Wildflowers, Spruce-fir	Great Views, Swimming, Photo Opportunity, Historic Interest, Steep
39	2	3.6	Point-to-Point	Dayhiking, Child Friendly	Summit, Ridgeline	Autumn Colors, Wildflowers, Spruce-fir	Great Views, Photo Opportunity

USES & ACCESS	TYPE	TERRAIN	FLORA & FAUNA	FEATURES
Dayhiking	Loop	Mountain	Autumn Colors	Great Views
Backpacking	Out & Back	Summit	Wildflowers	Photo Opportunity
Horses	Point-to-Point	Ridgeline	Wildlife	Backcountry Camping
Child Friendly	DIFFICULTY - 1 2 3 4 5 + less more	Stream	Spruce-fir	Swimming
		Waterfall	Old-growth	Secluded
		Lake		Steep
				Historic Interest
				Geologic Interest

Maps

For the Deep, Forney, and Noland Creeks area, here are the USGS 7.5-minute (1:24,000-scale) topographic quadrangles that you will need, listed in the order that you will need them as you hike along your route.

Trail 32: Noland Creek
Trail 33: Noland Creek
Trail 34: Bryson City, Clingmans Dome
Trail 35: Bryson City
Trail 36: Bryson City, Clingmans Dome, Smokemont
Trail 37: Clingmans Dome
Trail 38: Clingmans Dome, Silers Bald, Noland Creek
Trail 39: Clingmans Dome

Deep, Forney, and Noland Creeks Area

Newton Bald Loop 265

Head up the famed fishing waters of Deep Creek to a streamside camp beneath white pines. Next, climb to a backcountry campsite 5,000 feet high on Thomas Divide. Follow the quiet Thomas Divide Trail back to Deep Creek.

TRAIL 36

Backpacking, Horses
22.5 miles, Loop
Difficulty: 1 2 3 4 **5**

Fork Ridge Loop 273

This challenging backpack loop has major elevation changes. Explore spruce-fir ridges and camp near high-elevation streams. Descend beneath big spruce and yellow birch trees on Fork Ridge to junglelike Deep Creek. Climb to the Appalachian Trail with views from Mount Collins.

TRAIL 37

Backpacking, Horses
20.1 miles, Loop
Difficulty: 1 2 3 4 **5**

Forney Creek Loop 281

This tough but rewarding backpack involves numerous creek fords and an elevation change of more than 4,000 feet one-way! Travel Forney Ridge, passing Andrews Bald, to make Forney Creek. Ascend Forney Creek and visit Forney Creek Cascades on your return trip.

TRAIL 38

Backpacking, Horses
19.4 miles, Loop
Difficulty: 1 2 3 4 **5**

Andrews Bald 287

From the park's highest trailhead, explore the extraordinary spruce-fir forest community on the way to the meadow of Andrews Bald, resplendent with stunning views.

TRAIL 39

Dayhiking, Child Friendly
3.6 miles, Out & Back
Difficulty: 1 **2** 3 4 5

Goldmine Loop

Travel a seldom-trod area of the Smokies, finding forgotten chimneys of old homesites. Gain views of Fontana Lake and small streams that feed it. Several old roads and trails spur off the loop, luring budding historians.

Best Time

Summer is when Fontana Lake is at full pool, and best for swimming. During fall the trails are their driest. Open winter woods reveal old homesites most clearly and avail maximum solitude.

Finding the Trail

From the Oconaluftee Visitor Center, head south on Newfound Gap Road for 3.2 miles to US 19 in Cherokee, North Carolina. Turn right on US 19 and follow it 10 miles to Bryson City, North Carolina. Once in Bryson City, turn right at the courthouse and continue straight on Everett Street, which soon becomes Lakeview Drive. The parking area is 7.9 miles from the courthouse in Bryson City, at the end of Lakeview Drive.

Trail Description

The Goldmine Loop is an undiscovered gem of a dayhike in the Smoky Mountains. Along the way you will see pioneer homesites and a slice of Fontana Lake and journey through the tunnel on the Road to Nowhere. Several old roads and trails branch off the Goldmine Loop, so watch your direction.

TRAIL USE
Dayhiking, Horses,
  Backpacking

LENGTH
3.2 miles, 1½–2½ hours

VERTICAL FEET
-650/+650

DIFFICULTY
– 1 **2** 3 4 5 +

TRAIL TYPE
Loop

FEATURES
Stream
Lake
Autumn Colors
Wildflowers
Secluded
Swimming
Historic Interest

FACILITIES
None

241

With your back to the Lakeview Road parking area, ▶1 pick up the Tunnel Bypass Trail across Lakeview Road. The tunnel is to your right and will be your return route. Once on the single-track Tunnel Bypass Trail, briefly traipse through a mountain laurel and rhododendron thicket, and then climb to a small gap at 0.3 mile. Several faint abandoned trails converge here. Proceed straight through the gap under pine, oak, and hickory woodland dotted with flowering dogwood. Skirt a knob to arrive at another gap and a trail junction at 0.4 mile. ▶2 Here, the Tunnel Bypass Trail leaves right 1.2 miles for the Lakeshore Trail, avoiding a trip through the tunnel bisecting Tunnel Ridge. This loop heads left with the Goldmine Loop Trail on a modest ridge.

Turn left on the Goldmine Loop Trail, and descend the slim crest well above Fontana Lake. At 0.9 mile, curve left to find Tunnel Branch and an old roadbed. A homesite was likely just upstream, but is now under a tangle of briers. The moisture-loving forest of beech, black birch, and tulip trees is denser than on the ridgetop. Tunnel Branch flows downhill under a sea of rhododendron to meet its mother waters of Fontana Lake, formerly the free-flowing Tuckasegee River.

The old road turns away from Tunnel Branch and comes to Fontana Lake and the embayment

 Autumn Colors

 Secluded

Stream

The sites of homes, schools, and churches now lie under Fontana Lake.

TRAIL 32 Goldmine Loop Elevation Profile

of Goldmine Branch at 1.3 miles. ▶3 Rich woodland reflects off the still blue-green waters of the impoundment. When drawn down, the lake's exposed mud bottom impairs the scenery.

Intersect another old road. Funny thing about these pre-park, pre-dam roads—they'll take you right to the lake, where you can see that the road continues but is now underwater. A short trip left will take you to the lake, but the official Goldmine

≋ **Lake**

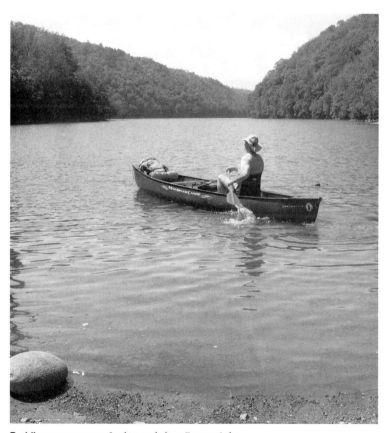

Paddlers can access *Smokies trails from Fontana Lake.*

Loop Trail veers right away from the lake to cross a tiny creek then cross Hyatt Branch. Span Goldmine Branch at 1.5 miles. Look for a small falls below the Goldmine Branch crossing. Judging by what the poor pioneers left behind, there was never any gold in these parts. Intersect the spur trail to Goldmine Branch Campsite, #67, at 1.6 miles. ▶4 The campsite is located at an open homesite a few hundred yards up the side trail and makes for a great one-night trip. Odds are you will have the campsite to yourself.

Resume a northbound, sometimes-muddy track astride small and shallow Goldmine Branch. Ahead, the trail briefly leaves the road and skirts to the right

▲ Backcountry Camping

Wildflowers

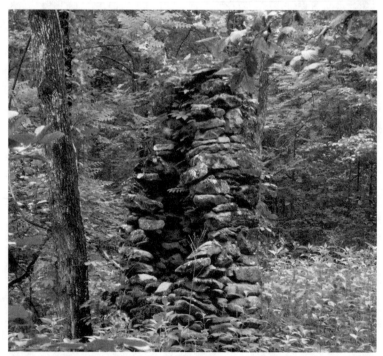

A crumbled chimney *is all that's left of this pioneer homestead along Goldmine Branch.*

of a homesite to rejoin the old road. The diminutive valley harbors a rhododendron tunnel under which you pass. Homesite clearings persist despite decades of park reforestation. A chimney stands mute near the path at 2.2 miles. ▶5 Consider the events that took place before that hearth.

Historic Interest

Swing past the homesite in another rhododendron tunnel to emerge atop the hollow. The old road continues straight but the Goldmine Loop makes a sharp right, heads uphill to a saddle, then veers left for a short but steep climb to meet the Lakeshore Trail at 2.5 miles. ▶6

Turn right on the Lakeshore Trail. Cruise easterly through oak woods, passing the other end of the Tunnel Bypass Trail. Keep forward to reach the Lakeview Road tunnel. Let your eyes adjust, and you can walk through it sans flashlight. Traverse the 0.2-mile long tunnel and emerge near the Lakeview Road and reach the trailhead. ▶7

⚐ MILESTONES

▶1	0.0	Lakeview Road Trailhead
▶2	0.4	Left on Goldmine Loop Trail
▶3	1.3	Fontana Lake
▶4	1.6	Spur trail to Goldmine Branch Campsite, #67
▶5	2.2	Trailside chimney
▶6	2.5	Right on Lakeshore Trail
▶7	3.2	Lakeview Road Trailhead

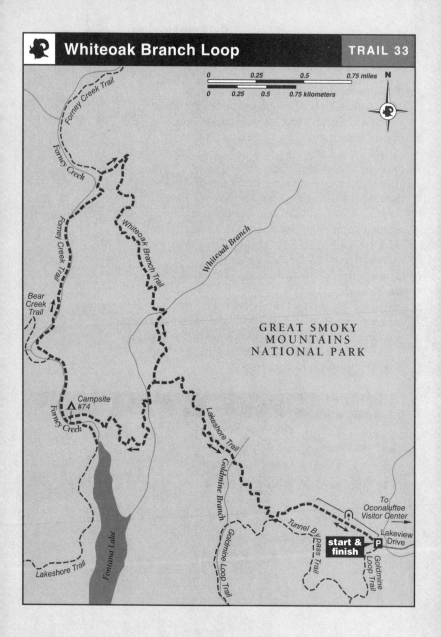

Whiteoak Branch Loop

Take the strange tunnel on the Road to Nowhere. Explore rushing lower Forney Creek and the still waters of Fontana Lake. Loop back through quiet woodlands once inhabited by North Carolina pioneers.

Best Time

Summer through early fall are the best time to enjoy the waters of Forney Creek. Plus it is when Fontana Lake is at its most scenic, at full pool. This is also when the trail and Fontana Lake are at their busiest as well. Solitude seekers will have this hike to themselves during cool to cold times.

Finding the Trail

From the Oconaluftee Visitor Center, head south on Newfound Gap Road for 3.2 miles to US 19 in Cherokee, North Carolina. Turn right on US 19 and follow it 10 miles to Bryson City, North Carolina. Once in Bryson City, turn right at the courthouse and continue straight on Everett Street, which soon becomes Lakeview Drive. The parking area is 7.9 miles from the courthouse in Bryson City, at the end of Lakeview Drive.

Trail Description

This hike offers a variety of landscapes—and waterscapes! Start your hike at Lakeview Road, also known as the Road to Nowhere. Follow a forsaken roadbed through a tunnel, and then trace the

TRAIL USE
Dayhiking, Horses
    Backpacking
LENGTH
8.8 miles, 5½–7 hours
VERTICAL FEET
+1,250/-1,250
DIFFICULTY
– 1 2 **3** 4 5 +
TRAIL TYPE
Loop

FEATURES
Ridgeline
Stream
Lake
Autumn Colors
Wildflowers
Historic Interest
Great Views
Swimming

FACILITIES
None

Lakeshore Trail to Gray Wolf Creek, where you begin the loop portion of the hike. Wander to lower Forney Creek, where the mountain cataract is at its largest and boldest before meeting the still waters of Fontana Lake. This watery impoundment bordering the south side of the park makes for a scenic setting where wooded ridges rise from translucent waters.

Your loop then leads upstream along Forney Creek, with its numerous cascades and pools beckoning a stop. All too soon, climb away from Forney to meet Whiteoak Branch. Here, traverse quiet ridges and small streamlets before returning to Gray Wolf Creek. Backtrack through the tunnel to the trailhead. Give yourself ample time to enjoy the hike as well as factor in stops at both Fontana Lake and Forney Creek. Although the elevation changes are never steep or long, repeated ups and downs add challenge to the hike.

Pick up the Lakeshore Trail ▶1 beyond the vehicle barriers on Lakeview Drive. Trace crumbling asphalt toward the tunnel, which stands in sight. You can stumble through the 0.2-mile tunnel without a flashlight; the light at the tunnel's end will guide you after your eyes adjust.

Emerge from the tunnel, and shortly the trail becomes a bona fide natural surface track bordered

This "Road to Nowhere" was promised to Swain County after Fontana Lake's creation, but it was halted because citizens didn't want a motorway cutting through the Smokies' south side.

TRAIL 33 Whiteoak Branch Loop Elevation Profile

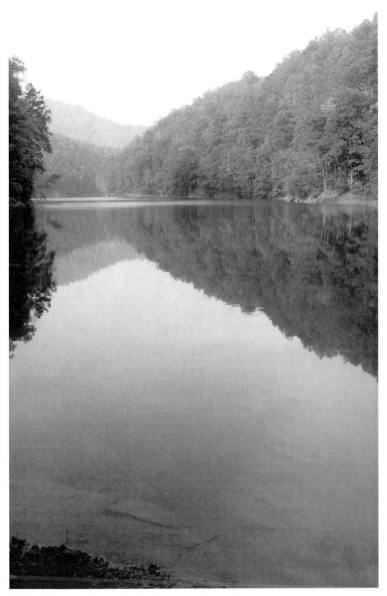

Still waters *on the Forney Creek embayment of Fontana Lake*

by pine, oak, and hickory forest with scads of mountain laurel. At 0.6 mile, the Tunnel Bypass Trail, ▶2 built mainly for horses (and people scared of hiking through tunnels), comes in on your left, having circled around Tunnel Ridge. At 0.7 mile, the Goldmine Loop Trail also comes in on your left. The Lakeshore Trail continues cruising hills and shallow drainages above Fontana Lake to meet Whiteoak Branch Trail in a homesite clearing at 2.0 miles. ▶3 You will return here later.

Stay left with the Lakeshore Trail, passing a spur road leading left, then bridging Gray Wolf Creek. Just beyond the bridge, a road to Woody Cemetery leads right, but the Lakeshore Trail curves left, southbound. Gray Wolf Creek crashes noisily below as you bisect a small gap then descend toward Forney Creek. Lower Forney backcountry campsite, #74, is visible just before reaching the Forney Creek Trail at 3.0 miles. ▶4 Turn left here, descending along the crashing stream. Bridge Forney Creek then reach Fontana Lake at 3.2 miles. ▶5 The slender Forney Creek embayment stretches south, bordered by rising tree-covered ridges. The confluence of the stream and lake lures boaters, anglers, and hikers, especially on summer weekends.

Backtrack to the Lakeshore Trail, resuming upstream along Forney Creek to meet the Bear Creek Trail at 3.8 miles. ▶6 Continue up Forney Creek Trail, looking for boulders to rest and sun yourself on along the way. The path leaves the stream at 4.7 miles, angling up the hillside in rhododendron to meet Whiteoak Branch Trail at 5.0 miles. ▶7 Turn right here, ascending along burbling Whiteoak Branch. Leave the trail's namesake watercourse, curving south, alternating between trickling branches in silent green coves and even quieter dry ridges, contrasting greatly with the roaring froth of Forney Creek. Meet the Lakeshore

Backcountry Camping

Lake

Stream

Wildflowers

Trail at 6.8 miles. ►8 Turn left here and backtrack 2 miles to the trailhead, ►9 once again passing through the strange tunnel at the end of the Road to Nowhere.

 Autumn Colors

🚶	**MILESTONES**	
►1	0.0	Lakeview Road Trailhead
►2	0.6	Pass Tunnel Bypass Trail
►3	2.0	Stay left on Lakeshore Trail
►4	3.0	Left on Forney Creek Trail with Lower Forney Campsite, #74
►5	3.2	Fontana Lake
►6	3.8	Pass Bear Creek Trail
►7	5.0	Right on Whiteoak Branch Trail
►8	6.8	Left on Lakeshore Trail
►9	8.8	Lakeview Road Trailhead

Indian Creek and Sunkota Ridge Loop

On this rewarding but long dayhike, pass two waterfalls and then walk along old homesteads amid riverine habitat of Indian Creek. Climb to Martins Gap and return via the quiet Sunkota Ridge Trail, with its drier forest.

Best Time

Winter offers maximum solitude and leafless woods, where you can see the homesites of Indian Creek more clearly. Spring presents wildflowers and the waterfalls at their boldest. Fall colors on Sunkota Ridge can be stunning. The trailhead and first 0.7 mile of the hike may be a madhouse in summer. The secluded part of the hike starts beyond this first 0.7 mile.

Finding the Trail

From the Oconaluftee Visitor Center, take US 441 south to Cherokee. Turn right on US 19 to Bryson City. Turn right at the Swain County Courthouse onto Everett Street, and carefully follow the signs through town to Deep Creek Campground. Inside the park, veer left toward the sign reading TRAIL-HEAD, WATERFALLS. The Deep Creek Trail starts shortly beyond the picnic area.

Alternate directions: From Exit 27 on I-40 west of Asheville, take US 74 west to the Bryson City exit. Once in Bryson City, follow the brown signs to Deep Creek Campground.

TRAIL USE
Dayhiking, Horses,
    Backpacking
LENGTH
12.0 miles, 6–7½ hours
VERTICAL FEET
+1,900/-1,900
DIFFICULTY
– 1 2 **3** 4 5 +
TRAIL TYPE
Loop

FEATURES
Ridgeline
Stream
Waterfall
Autumn Colors
Wildflowers
Secluded
Historic Interest

FACILITIES
Campground
Picnic tables
Restrooms
Water

Trail Description

You can appreciate the biological diversity of the Smokies on this valley and ridge trek. This circuit follows Deep Creek to Indian Creek, past Tom Branch Falls then Indian Creek Falls before you've gone a mile. Leave any crowds behind to climb to Martins Gap and return via the quiet Sunkota Ridge Trail, with its drier forest, then along Deep Creek and its accompanying riverine habitat.

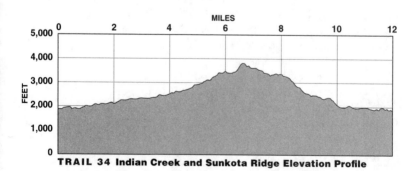

The Deep Creek Trail ►1 makes a wide track as it passes the spur trail to Juney Whank Falls. It reaches Tom Branch Falls at 0.2 mile. Tom Branch spills in four stages over rock slabs to fill Deep Creek, as Deep Creek in turn rushes over gray rocks, sometimes mossy, sometimes not, then slows in still pools. Bridge Deep Creek at 0.4 mile, just below an alluring pool.

Make the Indian Creek Trail junction at 0.7 mile. ►2 Turn right on the Indian Creek Trail, coming to Indian Creek Falls at 0.8 mile. ►3 A short side trail on your left leads to the base of the falls, which slopes 25 feet over a fanlike rock face into a large pool.

Gain a top-down view of Indian Creek Falls as you continue on up the trail, bridging Indian Creek at 0.9 mile. At 1.2 miles, the Stone Pile Gap Trail leaves right for Thomas Divide. ►4 This hike keeps

Stream

Waterfall

TRAIL 34 Indian Creek and Sunkota Ridge Elevation Profile

OPTIONS

Shorter, Easier Trek

For a much shorter and easier circuit of 3.2 miles, use the Loop Trail. Start this hike as described and at 1.5 miles, leave the Indian Creek Trail left on the Loop Trail, climbing 400 feet in a half mile to a gap on Sunkota Ridge. From here, continue tracing the Loop Trail downhill to the flat at Jenkins Place on Deep Creek. The wide Deep Creek Trail allows you to watch the delightful creek splash down the valley while you return to the trailhead.

up the moist valley amid everywhere-you-look beauty. Notice shiny mica rock at your feet. At 1.5 miles, the Loop Trail heads up Sunkota Ridge. ▶5

 Wildflowers

Stay north on the Indian Creek Trail. Look for remnants of clearings and nonnative trailside bushes. Locust and tulip trees are reclaiming the homesites. At 2.0 miles, bordering hills squeeze Indian Creek into a tight valley. At 2.2 miles, a spur trail leads to a pioneer cemetery. The valley widens again. At 2.9 miles, bridge Indian Creek. Bridge it again at 3.3 miles, then pass a second spur to another pioneer internment. At mile 3.6, bridge the creek again just before meeting the Deeplow Gap Trail. ▶6 *Bicycles are not allowed beyond this point.*

Historic Interest

Stream

Continue up Indian Creek, bridging it at 4.0, 4.3, and 4.5 miles to its end at 4.6 miles, in an old road turnaround near Estes Branch and backcountry campsite #46. ▶7

 Backcountry Camping

Here the park service arbitrarily starts the Martins Gap Trail. Cross now-smaller Indian Creek three times in a half mile on slim footbridges, before switchbacking up Sunkota Ridge. Arrive at Martins Gap, a sag on Sunkota Ridge, at 6.0 miles. ▶8 Turn left on the serene single-track Sunkota Ridge Trail.

A series of pioneer homesites appear on the creek sides.

Sunkota **is the pioneer**
interpretation of
the Cherokee word
meaning "apple."

Climb 450 feet to the loop's high point of 3,800 feet at 6.7 miles. ▶9 Begin a slow descent, winding along the ridgetop and its flanks. Enjoy your well-earned downgrade under oaks, maples, and pines. The higher Thomas Divide and Noland Divide are visible beyond the trees. A watery symphony from Indian Creek and Deep Creek drifts into your ears.

At 9.7 miles, meet the Loop Trail. ▶10 Turn right on the Loop Trail, descending to a flat and the old Jenkins Place, another pioneer homestead, to intersect Deep Creek Trail at 10.3 miles. ▶11 Follow the wide Deep Creek Trail downstream over three bridges to meet the Indian Creek Trail at 11.3 miles. ▶12 Return to the trailhead on the short section of the Deep Creek Trail you traversed earlier. Complete your loop at 12.0 miles. ▶13

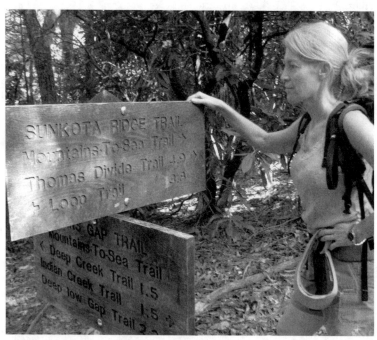

A hiker checks out *trail signs at Martins Gap.*

🚶 MILESTONES

▶1   0.0   Deep Creek Trailhead
▶2   0.7   Right on Indian Creek Trail
▶3   0.8   Indian Creek Falls
▶4   1.2   Pass Stone Pile Gap Trail
▶5   1.5   Pass Loop Trail
▶6   3.6   Pass Deeplow Gap Trail
▶7   4.6   Campsite #46, and join Martin Gap Trail
▶8   6.0   Martins Gap, and left on Sunkota Ridge Trail
▶9   6.7   High point of hike
▶10 9.7   Right on Loop Trail
▶11 10.3   Left on Deep Creek Trail at Jenkins Place
▶12 11.3   Pass Indian Creek Trail
▶13 12.0   Deep Creek Trailhead

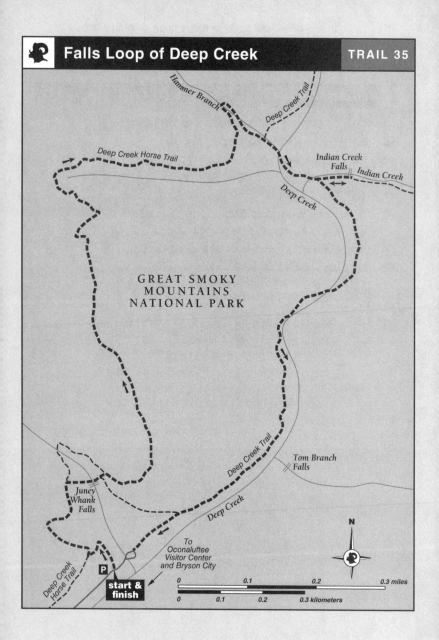

Hammer Branch

Deep Creek Trail

Deep Creek Horse Trail

Indian Creek Falls

Indian Creek

Deep Creek

GREAT SMOKY
MOUNTAINS
NATIONAL PARK

Deep Creek Trail

Tom Branch Falls

Juney Whank Falls

Deep Creek

To Oconaluftee Visitor Center and Bryson City

P

start & finish

Deep Creek Horse Trail

N

| 0 | 0.1 | 0.2 | 0.3 miles |
| 0 | 0.1 | 0.2 | 0.3 kilometers |

Falls Loop of Deep Creek

This great family dayhike has numerous rewards. Visit Juney Whank Falls, then cruise hills above Deep Creek before returning to visit cataract on Indian Creek. Enjoy a streamside cruise on lower Deep Creek, passing Tom Branch Falls.

TRAIL USE
Dayhiking,
   Child Friendly

LENGTH
2.4 miles, 1–2 hours

VERTICAL FEET
+390/-390

DIFFICULTY
– **1 2** 3 4 5 +

TRAIL TYPE
Loop

FEATURES
Stream
Waterfall
Autumn Colors
Wildflowers
Swimming
Photo Opportunity
Historic Interest

FACILITIES
Campground
Picnic tables
Water
Restrooms

Best Time

Winter and spring are best for seeing these waterfalls at their boldest. Also, you will find solitude then. Water lovers will want to come here during summer, but many others will enjoy the aquatic features with you then.

Finding the Trail

From the Oconaluftee Visitor Center, take US 441 south to Cherokee. Turn right on US 19 to Bryson City. Turn right at the Swain County Courthouse onto Everett Street and carefully follow the signs through town to Deep Creek campground. Inside the park, veer left toward signs reading TRAILHEAD, WATERFALLS. Juney Whank Falls Trail starts shortly at the upper end of the trail parking area before reaching the auto turnaround above the parking area.

Alternate directions: From Exit 27 on I-40 west of Asheville, take US 74 west to the Bryson City exit. Once in Bryson City, follow brown signs to Deep Creek Campground.

Trail Description

This hike begins at the developed Deep Creek area, ▶1 with its campground and picnic facilities, located on the park's edge near Bryson City. The Juney Whank Falls Trail leads uphill in rich woods, climbing along Juney Whank Branch. It isn't long before you reach the slender two-tier cataract that spills in a slender ribbon over a rock face, then under the trail before making a second dive toward Deep Creek.

Beyond here the hike wanders back to Deep Creek before it travels up another tributary, Indian Creek. Indian Creek Falls is a larger, wider waterfall that spills into a large pool. Next you return to Deep Creek, enjoying its everywhere-you-look beauty before coming to yet another tributary, Tom Branch. It makes a dramatic rocky plunge as it meets Deep Creek. A little more waterside walking returns you to the parking area.

Avoid this hike in the summertime if you disdain crowds. Lower Deep Creek can be crazy with tubers floating from the confluence of Indian Creek and Deep Creek through the Deep Creek Campground and beyond the park border.

The Juney Whank Falls Trail starts out as a wide gravel path leading from the parking area. Juney Whank Branch calmly flows to your right, after

TRAIL 35 Falls Loop of Deep Creek Elevation Profile

Tom Branch Falls *spills into Deep Creek.*

pouring off Beaugard Ridge. Shortly veer away from the watercourse, climbing to meet the Deep Creek Horse Trail at 0.1 mile. Watch for horses here, as a concessionaire operates nearby, using this route for a short distance. Stay right with the equestrian path in the second-growth woods of maple, pine, buckeye, beech, and tulip trees.

Reach the spur trail to Juney Whank Falls after a quarter mile. ▶2 Turn right here and descend a hill to reach a bridge and the falls. The low-flow cascade spills close enough to the bridge with a built-in observation deck and seat that you can nearly touch the water.

Leave Juney Whank Falls, rejoining the Deep Creek Horse Trail, after you pass a shortcut leading right, down to Deep Creek. Travel in pine-oak woods, turning up a quiet hollow. Dogwoods are plentiful here. The short tree with scaly brown bark and a widespread crown is easy to identify. It is widely regarded as one of the most beautiful trees in the Southeast. Dogwoods range from the eastern Texas north to Michigan, east to Massachusetts, and south to Florida. It grows in both moist and dry soils below 3,000 feet in the Smokies. In the spring dogwoods offers showy white or pinkish blooms. After greening up, dogwoods produce a shiny red fruit in fall. These small berrylike fruits taste bitter to humans but are an important food for birds. Dogwood is extremely hard and is used to make mallet heads, jeweler's blocks, and spools. The Cherokee used dogwood roots to make a red dye. Dogwoods growing in shady woods, such as these, are susceptible to a fungus known as dogwood anthracnose.

Reach a high point and a gap at 0.8 mile. ▶3 The Deep Creek Trail drifts toward Hammer Branch, following a trickling tributary. Curve to step over fast-flowing Hammer Branch, as a spur trail leaves for a pioneer cemetery. This hike then bridges Hammer Branch to meet the Deep Creek Trail at 1.4 miles. ▶4

▌ Waterfall

This waterfall is at its most dramatic during winter when it's frozen and spring when it flows strongest.

❀ Autumn Colors

Watch for bicycles in the next section, primarily during summer. Deep Creek flows broad and boisterous as you cross the stream on a wide bridge. Span Indian Creek to meet the Indian Creek Trail at 1.5 miles.

Historic Interest

Your second waterfall ▶5 stands a football field distant, up the Indian Creek Trail. An access path leads to the base of this broad, tumbling froth of whitewater. Indian Creek Falls plunges over a rock face into a pool open to the sky overhead. While here, grab a top-down view from the Indian Creek Trail, too.

Photo Opportunity

Your return trip leads down Deep Creek. The trail travels well above the creek, where you can look directly into the water. The path drops creekside then bridges Deep Creek. At 2.2 miles, reach your final fall. ▶2 Here, repose benches make a perfect observation point to see Tom Branch stairstep over a series of rock ledges, finally meeting Deep Creek. From here, your trip returns to the parking area after 0.2 mile. ▶7

Waterfall

🚶 MILESTONES

▶1	0.0	Deep Creek Trailhead
▶2	0.1	Deep Creek Horse Trail and Juney Whank Falls
▶3	0.8	High point at gap
▶4	1.4	Deep Creek Trail
▶5	1.6	Indian Creek Falls
▶6	2.2	Tom Branch Falls
▶7	2.4	Deep Creek Trailhead

Newton Bald Loop

TRAIL 36

N

0   0.5   1   1.5 miles
0   0.5   1   1.5 kilometers

Sunkota Ridge Trail

Newton Bald Trail

Campsite #54

Campsite #52

Pole Road Trail

Campsite #55

Deep Creek

Campsite #56

GREAT SMOKY MOUNTAINS NATIONAL PARK

Campsite #57

Thomas Divide Trail

Martins Gap Trail

Martins Gap Trail

Campsite #46

Campsite #58

Deeplow Gap Trail

Campsite #59

Sunkota Ridge Trail

Campsite #51

Deep Creek Trail

Indian Creek Motor Trail

Thomas Divide Trail

Campsite #60

Deep Creek

Indian Creek Trail

Indian Creek

Cooper Creek

Jenkins Place homesite

To Oconaluftee Visitor Center and Bryson City

cemetery

Indian Creek Falls

Stone Pile Gap Trail

Deep Creek Trail

Deep Creek Horse Trail

Tom Branch Falls

Thomas Divide Trail

P **start & finish**

Galbraith Creek Road

Newton Bald Loop

Head up the famed fishing waters of Deep Creek to a streamside camp beneath white pines. Next, climb to a backcountry campsite 5,000 feet high on Thomas Divide. Follow the quiet Thomas Divide Trail back to Deep Creek.

Best Time

Summer and early fall are ideal for fishing and swimming. Even during hot spells Deep Creek and Newton Bald will still be cool. Winter is a good option, too, since the trip requires no fords, even though it offers miles of streamside trekking in addition to high country action.

Finding the Trail

From the Oconaluftee Visitor Center, take US 441 south to Cherokee. Turn right on US 19 to Bryson City. Turn right at the Swain County Courthouse onto Everett Street, and carefully follow the signs through town to Deep Creek Campground. Inside the park, veer left following the sign reading, TRAIL-HEAD, WATERFALLS. The Deep Creek Trail starts shortly beyond the picnic area.

Alternate directions: From Exit #27 on I-40 west of Asheville, take US 74 west to the Bryson City exit. Once in Bryson City, follow brown signs to Deep Creek Campground.

TRAIL USE
Backpacking, Horses
LENGTH
22.5 miles,
   11–13½ hours
VERTICAL FEET
+3,100/-3,100
DIFFICULTY
− 1 2 3 4 **5** +
TRAIL TYPE
Loop

FEATURES
Ridgeline
Stream
Waterfall
Autumn Colors
Wildflowers
Wildlife
Swimming
Secluded
Historic Interest

FACILITIES
Campground
Picnic tables
Restrooms
Water

Trail Description

Enjoy an archetypal Smoky Mountain stream, and camp beside its singing waters. Next, loop into the high country and overnight at 5,000 feet on this two-night backpacking adventure. First you'll head up the famed waters of Deep Creek, where many a fishing exploit has taken place (then exaggerated about). Camp at a streamside site on a carpet of pine needles beneath a white pine grove.

Next, leave the Deep Creek watershed via the steep Martins Gap Trail. Hike Sunkota Ridge, where a ridgetop trek leads to little-used Newton Bald backcountry campsite on Thomas Divide. Finally, head south on Thomas Divide Trail back to Deep Creek, completing the circuit, but not before passing Indian Creek Falls.

Begin the hike on the wide Deep Creek Trail, ▶1 humming with hikers, bikers, and tubers in the summertime, to pass Tom Branch Falls at 0.2 mile. The tributary spills over rock ledges into Deep Creek. Pass the Indian Creek Trail junction at 0.7 mile. ▶2 Bridge Indian Creek and continue up Deep Creek Trail. The wide track continues upstream, crossing three bridges to meet the Loop Trail at the

---

Expect to see bear scat if not bears on Sunkota Ridge and Thomas Divide.

 Waterfall

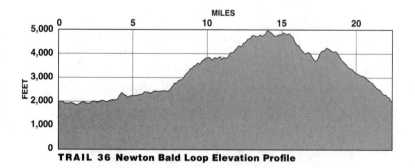

TRAIL 36 Newton Bald Loop Elevation Profile

Jenkins Place homesite at 1.7 miles. ▶3 The graded trail narrows some, and summertime crowds thin out. Wander alongside Deep Creek, which is following gravity's orders as it drains the Carolina side of Mount Collins, as well as the streams flowing down Noland Divide and Thomas Divide. Cross Bumgardner Branch, reaching Bumgardner Branch backcountry campsite, #60, at 2.9 miles. ▶4 Stay on the east bank of Deep Creek, rising far above the stream while surmounting Bumgardner Ridge. The creek sounds fade.

Backcountry Camping

Drop to McCracken Branch backcountry campsite, #59, at mile 4.2. ▶5 Repeat the pattern of rise and fall to make Nicks Nest Branch backcountry campsite, #58, at mile 5.5 ▶6 Trace the right bank of Deep Creek, coming to historic Bryson Place and the Martins Gap Trail, at 5.9 miles. ▶7 Once the site of a backwoods cabin and a hunting lodge, this piney place was a favorite haunt of famed outdoor writer and national park proponent Horace Kephart. Today, the locale is Bryson Place backcountry campsite, #57.

Backcountry Camping

Fishing continues to be a recreational pastime of many Smokies visitors. A monument to Mr. Kephart is just off the trail, on the Deep Creek side of the path before you reach the small stream at Bryson Place campsite. The monument spot was the location of Kephart's last camp in the Smokies before he perished in an automobile crash near Bryson City.

Historic Interest

Leave Bryson Place on the Deep Creek Trail and meet Burnt Spruce backcountry campsite, #56, elevation 2,405, at mile 6.2. ▶8 This is your first night's destination, under big white pines with Deep Creek rushing nearby. A wide streamside rock slab allows easy access to Deep Creek. Burnt Spruce campsite is situated between two campsites, Bryson Place and Pole Road, that receive heavier usage and thus remains a fine creekside camp.

Backcountry Camping

Day two begins by returning to Bryson Place, 0.3 mile back down Deep Creek Trail. ▶9 Turn left up the Martins Gap Trail, rising along a streamlet before bridging the watercourse. Wind up a galax-lined path under pines. Views of Deep Creek Valley open before you reach Martins Gap on Sunkota Ridge at mile 8.0 of your loop hike. ▶10 Turn left on infrequently trod single-track Sunkota Ridge Trail, gently ascending out of Martins Gap under oaks, maples, and sourwood. Pass a spring seep at 8.4 miles. Continue ascending, passing another seep at 9.2 miles. It seems the trail will top out, yet it keeps gaining elevation in moderate increments between gaps. Occasional glimpses of Noland Divide and Thomas Divide open beyond the trees. Break the 4,000-foot barrier at 10.4 miles, in a mix of oaks and northern hardwoods.

Intersect the Thomas Divide Trail at 12.5 miles. ▶11 It has come 4.6 miles from Newfound Gap Road. Turn right on the Thomas Divide Trail and walk 0.4 mile to arrive at Newton Bald Trail junction. Turn left on the Newton Bald Trail, ▶12 following it to Newton Bald backcountry campsite, #52, your second night's destination, at 13.0 miles. ▶13

This 5,000-foot-high campsite, located in a sag on Thomas Divide near what once was an open meadow, is a favorable place to escape the heat in summer and crowds anytime. During winter, Newton Bald campsite is susceptible to strong winds. Understory grasses are all that remain of the former meadow, which stretched easterly. Nowadays, white oaks, yellow birch, cherry, and red spruce shade the small camp. A cold, clear spring is accessed on a foot trail dropping off the east side of the gap, and is the headwaters of Cooper Creek.

Start day three by backtracking to the Thomas Divide Trail. ▶14 Turn left and begin a southwesterly course toward Deep Creek Campground on a lesser used path. Walk among wooded knolls

Secluded

Wildlife

Autumn Colors

Backcountry Camping

Secluded

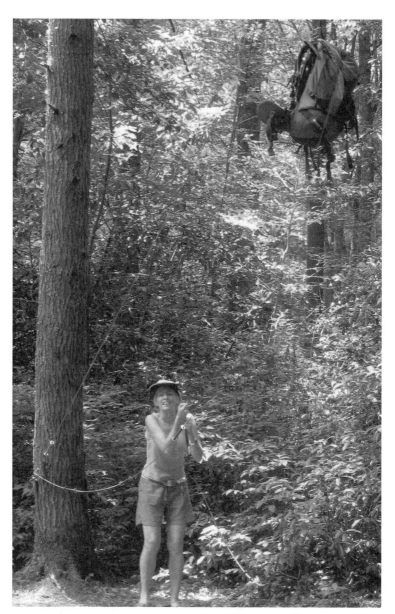

Food storage cables *such as this one at Campsite #56 keep backpackers' food safely stored.*

around 4,700-foot elevation for 1.5 miles, then begin a prolonged descent to reach Deeplow Gap and a trail junction at 16.0 miles of your loop hike. ►15 Climb out of Deeplow Gap, still on Thomas Divide Trail to soon pass a spring seep.

Autumn Colors

Top out at 17.0 miles. The downhill becomes relentless. Intersect the Indian Creek Motor Trail at 18.5 miles. ►16 The Thomas Divide Trail turns left here and traces a wide track that was originally designed to be an auto touring route. Public outcry stopped it in the late 1960s and early 1970s, but not before the route was graded for car use. Enjoy easy walking as you continually lose elevation. Meet the Stone Pile Gap Trail and the park boundary at 20.6 miles. ►17 Turn right here, back on single-track path, and continue your descent along a pine ridge, then repeatedly crisscross a small tributary of Indian Creek that often muddies the trail.

Waterfall

A footbridge leads over swift Indian Creek at 21.2 miles. Turn downstream to shortly intersect the Indian Creek Trail. ►18 Turn left onto the wide roadlike path open to bikes. Pass by Indian Creek Falls, ►19 a 25-foot cascade that fans over as rock slab into a mountain pool. Continue downhill to meet the Deep Creek Trail at 21.8 miles. ►20 Turn left on the Deep Creek Trail and follow it 0.7 mile to complete your backpacking circuit. ►21

MILESTONES

▶1	0.0	Deep Creek Trailhead
▶2	0.7	Stay left with Deep Creek Trail
▶3	1.7	Loop Trail leaves right
▶4	2.9	Bumgardner Branch Campsite, #60
▶5	4.2	McCracken Branch Campsite, #59
▶6	5.5	Nicks Nest Branch Campsite, #58
▶7	5.9	Bryson Place Campsite, #57, and Martins Gap Trail
▶8	6.2	Burnt Spruce Campsite, #56
▶9	6.5	Backtrack to reach Bryson Place Campsite, #57, and Martins Gap Trail
▶10	8.0	Reach Martins Gap, and left on Sunkota Ridge Trail
▶11	12.5	Right on Thomas Divide Trail
▶12	12.9	Left on Newton Bald Trail
▶13	13.0	Newton Bald Campsite, #52
▶14	13.1	Backtrack and turn left on Thomas Divide Trail
▶15	16.0	Pass Deeplow Gap Trail
▶16	18.5	Intersect Indian Creek Motor Trail, and stay left
▶17	20.6	Right on Stone Pile Gap Trail
▶18	21.3	Left on Indian Creek Trail
▶19	21.7	Indian Creek Falls
▶20	21.8	Left on Deep Creek Trail
▶21	22.5	Deep Creek Trailhead

Fork Ridge Loop

TRAIL 37

To Newfound Gap

start & finish

Clingmans Dome Road

Fork Ridge Trail

Sugarland Mountain Trail

441

Deep Creek

Deep Creek Trail

Collins Gap

Big Slick Ridge

Noland Divide Trail

GREAT SMOKY
MOUNTAINS
NATIONAL PARK

Campsite #53

Noland Creek

Bearpen Ridge

Roundtop Knob

Burnt Spruce Ridge

Deep Creek Trail

N

Pole Road Trail

Campsite #54

Deep Creek

0   0.25   0.5   0.75 miles
0 0.25 0.5 0.75 kilometers

Campsite #61

Noland Divide Trail

Sassafras Knob

Easy Ridge

Campsite #55

Campsite #56

Fork Ridge Loop

This challenging backpack loop has major elevation changes. Explore spruce-fir ridges and camp near high-elevation streams. Descend beneath big spruce and yellow birch trees on Fork Ridge to junglelike Deep Creek. Climb to the Appalachian Trail with views from Mount Collins.

Best Time

To access the trailhead Clingmans Dome Road must be open. This road, the park's highest, is generally open from April through November. Call ahead if you want to hike during the shoulder seasons. Midsummer through fall is best for fishing. Autumn offers color, solitude, and drier trails.

Finding the Trail

From Newfound Gap, take Clingmans Dome Road for 3.5 miles, to the Fork Ridge Trailhead, which will be on your left.

Trail Description

Enjoy highland stream camping along with many miles of rare spruce-fir forest. You will also experience ample solitude on this elevation-changing weekend loop. Take Fork Ridge Trail and amble beneath big spruce and yellow birch trees. Descend through transitioning forest types before reaching Deep Creek Valley and Poke Patch backcountry campsite. Poke Patch is not nearly as notable as the big trees, but it will do. Keep descending in attractive

TRAIL USE
Backpacking, Horses

LENGTH
20.1 miles, 12–14 hours

VERTICAL FEET
-4,300/+4,300

DIFFICULTY
– 1 2 3 4 **5** +

TRAIL TYPE
Loop

FEATURES
Ridgeline
Stream
Autumn Colors
Wildflowers
Spruce-fir
Great Views
Swimming
Steep
Secluded

FACILITIES
None

Deep Creek Valley to reach the Pole Road Creek Trail. *Note that the bridge over Deep Creek periodically washes out; ask about its status when you get your permit.* Climb to Noland Divide, only to drop to Noland Creek, and Bald Creek campsite. It requires a reservation, so call ahead for your permit. On the final day, backtrack to Noland Divide, then climb into evergreens near Clingmans Dome Road. Follow the road a short piece to intersect the Appalachian Trail, then trace the AT over Mount Collins. Enjoy the view from 6,000-plus feet before completing the loop.

Start the overnight loop ▶1 on the single-track hiker-only Fork Ridge Trail. This trail is also part of North Carolina's Mountains-to-Sea Trail, which accounts for the circular white blazes. Cruise a narrow path where sturdy old-growth red spruce hold sway overhead, complemented by yellow birch, Fraser fir, and ferns aplenty. Partial vistas open to the east. Curve toward a feeder stream of Keg Drive Branch at 1.6 miles. The stream was named for Cherokee hunter Jim Keg. As the trail drops, cherry, beech, and other deciduous trees rise in the forest. Giant trailside hemlock trunks still stand, waiting for a big storm to blow them down.

Rejoin the slender ridgecrest at 2.6 miles. Dry environment species, such as chestnut oak, sourwood, and mountain laurel, appear. Views into Left

Secluded

Old-growth

Autumn Colors

TRAIL 37 Fork Ridge Loop Elevation Profile

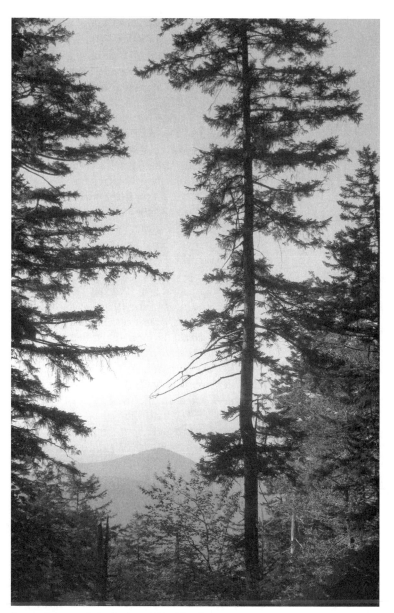

Spruce trees *reach for the sky on Noland Divide.*

Fork Deep Creek open. Fork Ridge is the divide between the forks of Deep Creek. The sounds of both forks drift upward on your downgrade. Reach Deep Creek Gap at 4.6 miles. ►2 The trail makes an abrupt left turn and plunges toward Deep Creek on a sheer slope. Just before reaching Deep Creek, look left at a switchback for a faint trail leading left 40 yards to a huge tulip tree. The circumference of this ancient poplar will amaze you.

Return to the main trail and soon come to Deep Creek. This is usually a wet crossing. Just across the stream, at 5.2 miles, is the junction with the Deep Creek Trail and the Poke Patch backcountry campsite, #53. ►3 The camping flat, open to the sky overhead, has been used for a long time and shows signs of wear. This is your first night's destination.

Start the second day by heading downstream on the Deep Creek Trail, laid out by the Civilian Conservation Corps in the 1930s. Walk beneath a cathedral of more large trees. Rhododendron and doghobble create an incredibly dense eye-level cavalcade of greenery. Deep Creek is sometimes seen, but always heard. At mile 5.9 of your loop hike, step over Cherry Creek. Climb away from the stream, only to drop directly alongside Deep Creek among rocks. The trail here was blasted out of the mountainside to avoid a ford. Beetree Creek falls in from your left at 6.3 miles. Wind deeper into luxuriant Deep Creek Valley to reach Nettle Creek and backcountry campsite #54 at mile 7.5. ►4 Beyond this campsite, sycamores appear in the forest. Open to a flat rife with white pines, reaching Pole Road backcountry campsite, #55, with a horse-hitching rack and picnic tables, at mile 8.5. ►5

Intersect the Pole Road Creek Trail just ahead. Cross Deep Creek on a footbridge high above Deep Creek. ►6 *This bridge periodically washes out through the years and is then replaced. When obtaining your backcountry permit, ask about the bridge's status.* Soon

A Backcountry Camping

R Stream

✳ Wildflowers

A Backcountry Camping

A Backcountry Camping

step over Pole Road Creek. When the Deep Creek Valley was selectively logged, timber men placed poles at intervals to slide felled trees down Pole Road Creek Valley to Deep Creek where they were amassed at splash dams, then floated downstream after heavy rains.

Cross Pole Road Creek at 9.4 miles. The trail steepens a bit and crosses the stream again at miles 9.7, 10.0, and 10.1. Pass a huge tulip tree just before the final crossing at 10.6 miles. ▶7 Swing around a rib ridge of Noland Divide. Easterly views open amid naked dead hemlocks. Keep ascending in oaks and mountain laurel to reach Upper Sassafras Gap on Noland Divide at mile 11.8. ▶8

 Steep

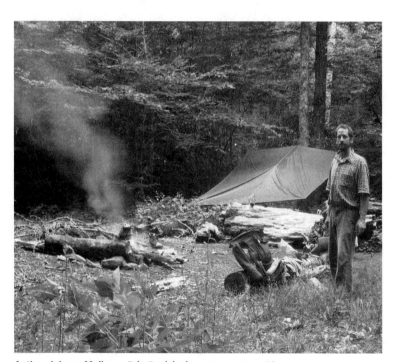

Author Johnny Molloy *at Poke Patch backcountry campsite, #53*

Catch your breath at the gap, then drop into rhododendron, now on the Noland Creek Trail. The roar of Noland Creek hastens your step. Watch for views of nearby Forney Ridge. Reach Noland Creek then turn downstream to meet Bald Creek Campsite, #61, at mile 12.8. ▶9 This two-tiered campsite is your second night's destination.

Start day three by backtracking to Noland Divide, reaching Upper Sassafras Gap at mile 13.8 ▶10 of your loop hike. Turn left in an oak forest on the Noland Divide Trail, and begin a steady uptick to a small knob. Catch your breath in rhododendron thickets on a level stretch at 14.5 miles. Circle Roundtop Knob to level out at 5,200 feet at 15.8 miles.

Stair-step in primeval spruce, fir, and yellow birch woodland to reach a grassy road at mile 17.0. ▶11 This closed road accesses a water source and acid rain–monitoring stations, one of which you pass. Reach Clingmans Dome Road at mile 17.5. ▶12 Turn right here and descend Clingmans Dome Road for 0.7 mile. Dip left into the woods, reaching the Appalachian Trail at Collins Gap. If you come to a parking area on the right with 11 spaces in it, you have gone a little too far.

Once on the AT, turn right, northbound. ▶13 Climb 500 feet from Collins Gap and over Mount Collins, reaching 6,188 feet and a Carolina view at 19.5 miles. ▶14 Drop to intersect Sugarland Mountain Trail at mile 19.9. ▶15 Stay on the AT and intersect Fork Ridge Connector Trail at mile 20.1. ▶16 Turn right here, and walk a few steps to Clingmans Dome Road, completing your loop.

Great Views

🚶 MILESTONES

▶1   0.0   Fork Ridge Trailhead
▶2   4.6   Left at Deep Creek Gap
▶3   5.2   Poke Patch Campsite, #53
▶4   7.5   Nettle Creek Campsite, #54
▶5   8.5   Pole Road Creek Campsite, #55
▶6   8.6   Cross Deep Creek on Pole Road Creek Trail
▶7   10.6   Leave Pole Road Creek
▶8   11.8   Upper Sassafras Gap, and descend Noland Creek Trail
▶9   12.8   Bald Creek Campsite, #61
▶10 13.8   Upper Sassafras Gap, and left on Noland Divide Trail
▶11 17.0   Reach a grassy roadbed
▶12 17.5   Right on Clingmans Dome Road
▶13 18.2   Join AT northbound from Collins Gap
▶14 19.5   View into Carolinas from atop Mount Collins
▶15 19.9   Pass Sugarland Mountain Trail
▶16 20.1   Right on Fork Ridge Connector to reach trailhead

Forney Creek Loop **TRAIL 38**

To Newfound Gap

Clingmans Dome

Clingmans Dome Road

TENNESSEE
NORTH CAROLINA

Clingmans Dome Bypass Trail

start & finish

P

Forney Ridge Trail

Takessah Ridge

Loggy Ridge

Steeltrap Creek

Suli Knob

GREAT SMOKY MOUNTAINS NATIONAL PARK

Forney Creek

Andrews Bald

Firescald Ridge

Suli Ridge

Clingmans Dome Vista

Forney Ridge Trail

Jonas Creek

Huggins Creek

ford

ford

Huggins Campsite #69

massive oak

Buckhorn Bald

Forney Ridge

ford

ford

Jonas Creek Campsite #70

White Oak Ridge

Board Camp Gap

Springhouse Branch Trail

Noland Creek Trail

CCC Campsite #71

Forney Creek

Bee Gum Branch

N

0   0.5   1   1.5 miles

0   0.5   1   1.5 kilometers

Forney Creek Loop

This tough but rewarding backpack involves numerous creek fords and an elevation change of more than 4,000 feet one-way! Travel Forney Ridge, passing Andrews Bald, to make Forney Creek. Ascend Forney Creek and visit Forney Creek Cascades on your return trip.

Best Time

To access the trailhead Clingmans Dome Road must be open. This road, the park's highest, is generally open from April through November. Call ahead if hiking the shoulder seasons. June features great rhododendron and flame azalea blooms. Midsummer through fall is best for swimming and fishing Forney Creek. Fording the streams is safer then because the waterways are at their lowest.

Finding the Trail

From Newfound Gap, drive 7 miles to the end of Clingmans Dome Road. The Forney Ridge Trail starts at the southwestern end of the Clingmans Dome parking area, just before the parking area loop road curves away from Clingmans Dome.

Trail Description

This is a tough but rewarding two-night backpack, involving numerous creek fords, an elevation change of more than 4,000 feet, and a long first day. Leave Clingmans Dome and travel Forney Ridge, passing Andrews Bald with its wonderful views.

TRAIL USE
Backpacking, Horses
LENGTH
19.4 miles, 11–13 hours
VERTICAL FEET
-4,200/+4,200
DIFFICULTY
- 1 2 3 4 **5** +
TRAIL TYPE
Loop

FEATURES
Ridgeline
Stream
Waterfall
Autumn Colors
Wildflowers
Spruce-fir
Great Views
Historic Interest
Swimming
Steep
Photo Opportunity

FACILITIES
Water
Restrooms
Bookstore

Continue down Forney Ridge to reach the Civilian Conservation Corps campsite on Forney Creek. You must have a reservation to stay at CCC backcountry campsite, #71; call (865) 436-1231 to reserve a spot. Turn up Forney Creek, ascending a wild valley along a scintillating mountain stream capped with a visit to Forney Creek Cascades, one of the best rock slides in the entire Southern Appalachians.

Along Forney Creek, logging and settler relics can be spotted by observant hikers. Remember to leave artifacts for others to discover and enjoy. Be apprised that Forney Creek Trail has several fords, which are challenging at high water. For your second night's destination of Steeltrap campsite, camp in a lesser-used clearing or beside Forney Creek Cascades. Your final day climbs back into the spruce-fir high country.

Leave Clingmans Dome parking area ►1 on the Forney Ridge Trail, bordered by big boulders, Fraser fir, and mountain ash. Bear left after meeting the Clingmans Dome Bypass Trail. The rough, rocky track winds in and out of shade. Open areas allow southwesterly views. Spruce and fir grow in dense thickets elsewhere, along with yellow birch. Meet the Forney Creek Trail, your return route, at 1.1 miles. ►2 At 1.8 miles, open onto the upper

A Great Views

TRAIL 38 Forney Creek Loop Elevation Profile

end of Andrews Bald. ▶3 Blueberries, azaleas, and **Wildflowers**
rhododendron bushes dot the meadow, which avails
views south to Fontana Lake and waves of Carolina
mountains beyond.

Beyond the bald, the trail receives much less use.
Work downhill, under partial tree canopy. Brambles
and briars crowd the path during summertime.
Occasional spinelike rock protrusions emerge from
the trailside. At 3.1 miles, while curving around a
knob, a view of Clingmans Dome opens to the right.
Keep descending, leaving the high country ever-
greens, now in oak woods. The trail rambles either ▲ **Ridgeline**
the crest or the right-hand side of Forney Ridge
while trending downhill amid occasional pockets of
rhododendron.

In a gap, at 4.5 miles, the trail passes a massive
oak tree. From here, the Forney Ridge Trail gently
undulates beneath now-wooded Buckhorn Bald.
Make Board Camp Gap and join the Springhouse
Branch Trail at 5.8 miles. ▶4 The junction is a nice
place for a break, with a level area and trees against
which to lean. From Board Camp Gap, the trail
undulates on a narrow wooded ridge, then makes
a hard switchback right at 7.1 miles, ▶5 leaving
Forney Ridge. Wind in and out of hollows, crossing the headwaters of Bee Gum Branch at 7.7 miles.
Keep westerly in this valley, staying well above Bee
Gum Branch, alternately entering moist hollows and
drier mountain laurel, oak, and sassafras woods.

You keep hearing water, thinking you're almost
there. Make a couple of last switchbacks then **Backcountry**
open onto CCC Campsite, #71, elevation 2,160 feet, **Camping**
at 9.9 miles. ▶6 This former homesite and Civilian
Conservation Corps Camp has a large chimney and
metal artifacts. The CCC boys who built the trail 🏠 **Historic Interest**
you just walked were headquartered here. This
busy campsite, open to hikers and equestrians, is
your first night's destination. Forney Creek rumbles
nearby, providing fishing and swimming venues. **Swimming**

Follow the railroad grade upstream from the camp to an old stone trestle at the creek's edge. There you will find two large pools.

Start your 6-mile second day, turning up Forney Creek Trail as it veers away from the stream to avoid fords, then descends to reach a former logging railroad grade, at 10.7 miles of your loop hike. The trail becomes quite rocky before intersecting the Jonas Creek Trail at 11.1 miles. ▶7 Jonas Creek back country campsite, #70, is across the bridge from the Forney Creek Trail. The Forney Creek Trail is open only to hikers from this point forward. Continue up the lush valley bordered by doghobble, mountain laurel, and rhododendron, passing through huge forested flats.

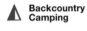
Backcountry Camping

Make ford #1 and ford #2 of Forney Creek at 11.6 miles and 12.1 miles. These are wet fords under normal flows, though late summer and fall may allow a nimble rock-hopper dry passage. Continue up the right bank, reaching ford #3 and Huggins Campsite, #69, at 12.4 miles. ▶8 This backcountry campsite was historically known as Monteith Camp. Metal logging relics lie about. After ford #4, just beyond Huggins, the trailbed becomes wet and rocky. Switchback past an enormous rock retaining wall, left over from the railroad days. The trail is well above the stream after making another switchback.

Backcountry Camping

Reach ford #5 at 14.0 miles. This crossing takes you to the left-hand bank. More switchbacks lie ahead, entering great cove hardwood forests where tulip trees grow straight and tall. This railroad grade was made gentle enough for tree-loaded flatcars to ascend these mountains; therefore, a backpacker loaded with camping gear should be able to make it as well.

Reach lower Steeltrap Campsite, #68B, at 15.9 miles, ▶9 a short ways after stepping over Steeltrap Creek. A clearing has a single fire ring. Upper

Steeltrap Campsite, #68A, elevation 4,250 feet. #68B, is up the trail 0.4 mile at 16.3 miles, ▶**10** near Forney Creek Cascades. That site has old railroad artifacts including wheels and rail. The cascades are a wide rock slide about 50 to 60 feet high, with another fall above it. Interestingly, quartz striations run through the cascade rocks. Either campsite is your second night's destination.

Start your 3-mile third day by crossing uppermost Forney Creek one last time, an easy step over. Railroad artifacts continue amid a northern hardwood forest of beech, sugar maple, and yellow birch. Spruce and fir trees mix in as you climb. Curve into a watery rock garden, making a big switchback away from the water. Ascend a wet rocky track, making a last hard switchback to the right before reaching the Forney Ridge Trail at 18.3 miles. ▶**11** From here, backtrack 1.1 miles to Clingmans Dome, ▶**12** completing your two-night backpack loop.

 Backcountry Camping

 Historic Interest

 Waterfall

 Spruce–Fir

 Steep

MILESTONES

▶1	0.0	Clingmans Dome Trailhead
▶2	1.1	Straight on Forney Ridge Trail
▶3	1.8	Andrews Bald
▶4	5.8	Join Springhouse Branch Trail at Board Camp Gap
▶5	7.1	Leave Forney Ridge on hard switchback
▶6	9.9	Reach CCC campsite, #71
▶7	11.1	Pass Jonas Creek Trail
▶8	12.4	Huggins Campsite, #69
▶9	15.9	Lower Steeltrap Campsite, #68B
▶10	16.3	Upper Steeltrap Campsite, #68A
▶11	18.3	Left on Forney Ridge Trail
▶12	19.4	Clingmans Dome Trailhead

Andrews Bald

TRAIL 39

GREAT SMOKY
MOUNTAINS
NATIONAL PARK

To
Newfound
Gap

Clingmans Dome Bypass

Clingmans Dome Trail

Clingmans Dome Road

Forney Creek

P

start & finish

Forney Creek Trail

Forney Ridge Trail

N

Andrews
Bald

0   0.1   0.2   0.3 miles

0   0.1   0.2   0.3 kilometers

Andrews Bald

From the park's highest trailhead, explore the extraordinary spruce-fir forest community on the way to the meadow of Andrews Bald, resplendent with stunning views.

Best Time

To access the trailhead Clingmans Dome Road must be open. This road, the park's highest, is generally open from April through November. Call ahead if hiking the shoulder seasons. June features great Catawba rhododendron blooms, as well as flame azaleas. August is good for blueberry picking, and fall is best for views. In midsummer the bald is sometimes enshrouded in fog and mist.

Finding the Trail

From Newfound Gap, drive 7 miles to the end of Clingmans Dome Road. The Forney Ridge Trail starts at the southwestern end of the Clingmans Dome parking area, just before the parking area loop road curves away from Clingmans Dome.

Trail Description

This is one of the Smokies' finest hikes. The trip passes through an extraordinary spruce-fir forest to the grassy field of Andrews Bald. Resplendent with stunning views, the mountain meadow is the ideal backdrop for a picnic in the sky. The origin of these fields is not clear, although natural fires, clearing by Indians, and grazing cattle possibly kept

TRAIL USE
Dayhiking,
   Child Friendly

LENGTH
3.6 miles, 1½–2½ hours

VERTICAL FEET
-600/+150

DIFFICULTY
– 1 **2** 3 4 5 +

TRAIL TYPE
Out & Back

FEATURES
Summit
Ridgeline
Autumn Colors
Wildflowers
Spruce-fir
Great Views
Photo Opportunity

FACILITIES
Water
Restrooms
Bookstore

the fields clear. Balds once stretched along many ridges in the Smokies and throughout the Southern Appalachians. In summer, residents of the nearby lowlands would drive their cattle up to these balds to graze, which certainly helped keep the balds open; when the practice ceased trees began reclaiming the meadows. Now, only names recall the balds of the Smokies, save for this one and Gregory Bald. Outside the park, on nearby lands, national forests are keeping other balds open.

Those who want to restore the Southern Appalachians to their "original" state find the question about preserving the balds a vexing one. Are the historic vistas worth keeping, or should they keep the balds for their natural qualities? Or allow them to disappear? Hikers are lured to the balds. Most are glad the balds are kept open. Views in this verdant, mountainous forest are limited.

After leaving the busy Clingmans Dome parking area ▶1 on the Forney Ridge Trail, descend a gravel track bordered by boulders to reach a trail junction at 0.1 mile. The Clingmans Dome Bypass Trail heads right, but you stay left with the Forney Ridge Trail, which drops along a rocky section that allows views to the south. Closed-in areas are inhabited by an evergreen forest reminiscent of Maine or Canada.

Andrews Bald is one of only two grassy fields in the Smokies that the park service maintains in their open state.

 Great Views

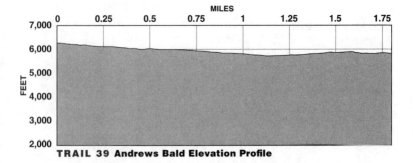

TRAIL 39 Andrews Bald Elevation Profile

The smell of red spruce and Fraser fir waft into your nostrils while northern red squirrels, also known as boomers, scold you from cone-laden green boughs. This area receives upward of 90 inches of rain per year, and the trail is built with water bars of stone and wood, along with steps and even boardwalks, to minimize erosion and allow hikers to focus on the unique surroundings. At 1.1 miles, intersect the Forney Creek Trail. ▶2 It leads right and downhill 10-plus miles to Fontana Lake.

🌲 Spruce–Fir

This hike continues along the undulating and rocky Forney Ridge to arrive at the northern end of Andrews Bald at mile 1.8. ▶3 The highland meadow, dotted with bushes and occasional trees, stands at an elevation of 5,800 feet. The lush grass beckons you to lie down, letting the sweat dry off. But that would deny you the expansive views of the southern range of the Smokies and beyond, as far south as the clarity of the sky allows. Fontana Lake is plainly visible on a clear day. Cool breezes drift in from the woods, countering a warm summer sun. This bald, the Smokies' highest, offers marvelous flower displays in June, and blueberries and blackberries in late summer.

🔺 Ridgeline

Andrews Bald was historically known as Anders Bald until an errant mapmaker renamed it Andrews Bald, which stuck.

Trees border the meadow as it drops off Forney Ridge, and the Forney Ridge Trail disappears into the woods, aiming for Forney Creek. Most hikers find a grassy seat and enjoy the scene before backtracking to the Clingmans Dome Trailhead.

🚶 **MILESTONES**

▶1	0.0	Clingmans Dome Trailhead
▶2	1.1	Straight on Forney Ridge Trail
▶3	1.8	Andrews Bald

Smokemont, Cataloochee, and Big Creek Area

Smokemont, Cataloochee, and Big Creek Area

Smokemont, Cataloochee, and Big Creek together comprise the most easterly North Carolina section of the park. Top to bottom it contains some of the highest terrain in the entire park. Newfound Gap Road and the Oconaluftee River form the western boundary of the area. The state line ridge dividing North Carolina and Tennessee creates the northern border. On this crest, elevations remain above 5,000 feet for more than 20 miles. Spruce-fir forests cloak this division between the states. Evergreens also run atop spur ridges, including high and wild Balsam Mountain. Balsam Mountain roughly divides Smokemont from Cataloochee and Big Creek.

Several big streams drain southward from the mountain crests. The streams west of Balsam Mountain—Oconaluftee River and Raven Fork—flow beyond the park and through the adjacent Cherokee Indian Reservation and into the Tuckasegee River. The streams east of Balsam Mountain—Cataloochee Creek and Big Creek—pour into the Pigeon River.

Elevations range from higher than 6,500 feet along the state line ridge and Appalachian Trail to 1,600 feet where Big Creek exits the park. However, the area is far more high elevation than not and has the highest average elevation of any park segment. Most of these highest points remained wild until the park was established. The lowest elevations, primarily Bradley Fork, a tributary of the Oconaluftee River, and the lower Cataloochee Valley, were settled by pioneers, but much of this was Indian country. The ultrarugged Raven Fork valley was where many Cherokees hid during the westward Indian removal of the 1830s. The remaining band then successfully petitioned to have a reservation. It now borders the park.

Cataloochee is a bucolic valley tucked away in the southeastern corner of the park. It is home to pioneer settler structures as well as wild elk that roam

Overleaf and opposite: Evergreens rise *near and far from the perch atop Mount Sterling (Trail 49).*

green meadows from which rise the great mountaintop evergreen forests. Although lower Big Creek was headquarters for a lumber operation, the forest has regrown to such a state that most visitors can't tell it was ever logged. Big Creek, a gorgeous mountain stream with big boulders and big pools, is a gateway for entering the spruce-fir forest that virtually encircles it.

There are plenty of loop hikes in this area, thanks to a favorable trail network. These loops range from shorter dayhikes to overnight backpacks. If you like streams, there is plenty of waterside walking, miles and miles of it. But this is also where hikers can and should explore the high country. One major reason: These high ridges exhibit the same characteristics as the state line ridge upon which the busy Appalachian Trail travels. Here, you can enjoy high country ridge walking in solitude. Flat Creek Falls and Vista, Trail 43, combines high country vistas with one of the highest elevation streams in the park.

Smokemont, Cataloochee, and Big Creek each have a primary trailhead at their respective campgrounds. Balsam Mountain Campground is accessed off the Blue Ridge Parkway. Each campground has at least one hike nearby campers can enjoy. Numerous other entry points exist, and the hikes here take advantage of them. Highlights of this area are historic—pioneer homes and churches of Cataloochee, for instance. They are also watery—Chasteen Creek Cascades, Gunter Fork Falls, and Mouse Creek Falls. They are natural—the Big Poplars—huge old-growth tulip trees, miles of spruce-fir atop Balsam Mountain, and majestic Mount Sterling. And they are eye opening: the extensive views from Hemphill Bald and a 360-degree vista from the historic fire tower atop Mount Sterling.

Permits

Permits are *not* required for dayhiking. Backpackers, however, must get a backcountry permit to stay at one of the 15 designated backcountry campsites and trail shelters located in this area. About half the campsites require a simple self-registration; however, others require a reservation, which you can make by calling the backcountry permit office at (865) 436-1231. Pick up and fill out backcountry permits at the Smokemont Campground entrance station, in Cataloochee Valley near the campground, at Big Creek Ranger Station, and at the Oconaluftee Visitor Center.

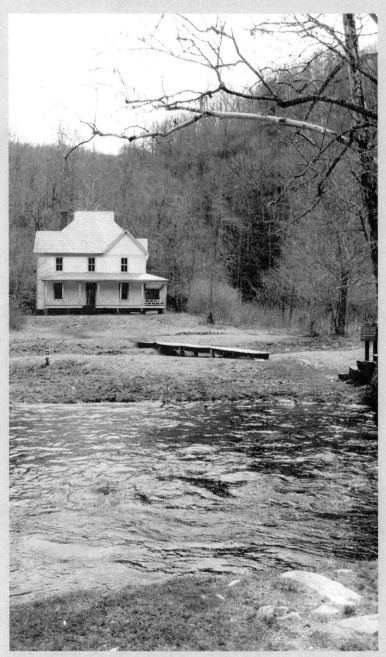

The Woody Place *(Trail 45) on Rough Fork in Cataloochee*

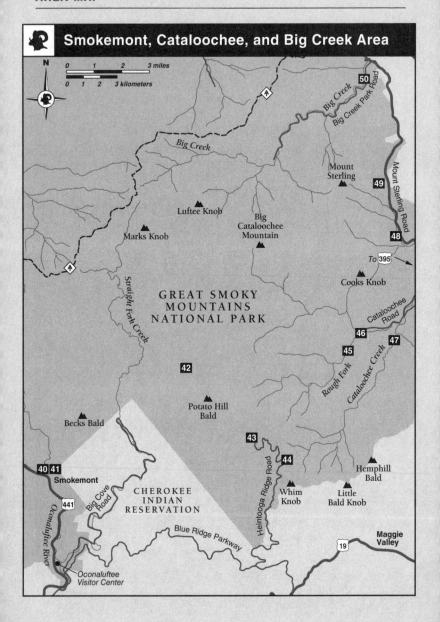

Smokemont, Cataloochee, and Big Creek Area

N

0   1   2   3 miles

0   1   2   3 kilometers

Big Creek

50

Big Creek Park Road

Big Creek

Mount Sterling Road

Mount Sterling

49

Luftee Knob

Big Cataloochee Mountain

48

Marks Knob

To 395

Cooks Knob

GREAT SMOKY MOUNTAINS NATIONAL PARK

Straight Fork Creek

Cataloochee Road

46

45

47

42

Rough Fork

Cataloochee Creek

Potato Hill Bald

Becks Bald

43

44

Hemphill Bald

40 41

Smokemont

441

Big Cove Road

CHEROKEE INDIAN RESERVATION

Heintooga Ridge Road

Whim Knob

Little Bald Knob

Oconaluftee River

Blue Ridge Parkway

19

Maggie Valley

Oconaluftee Visitor Center

Smokemont, Cataloochee, and Big Creek Area

TRAIL	Difficulty	Length	Type	USES & ACCESS	TERRAIN	FLORA & FAUNA	OTHER
40	2	6.0	Loop	Dayhiking	Stream, Summit, Mountain	Autumn Colors, Wildflowers	Great Views, Secluded
41	4	17.4	Loop	Backpacking, Horses	Stream, Waterfall, Mountain	Autumn Colors, Wildflowers	Swimming, Historic Interest
42	3	7.6	Loop	Dayhiking, Horses	Stream, Mountain	Autumn Colors, Wildflowers	Secluded, Steep
43	2	3.8	Out & Back	Dayhiking, Child Friendly	Stream, Waterfall, Mountain	Autumn Colors, Spruce-fir	Great Views, Photo Opportunity
44	3–4	9.6	Out & Back	Backpacking	Mountain	Autumn Colors, Wildflowers, Spruce-fir	Great Views, Photo Opportunity, Secluded
45	3	9.1	Loop	Dayhiking, Backpacking, Horses	Stream, Mountain	Autumn Colors, Wildflowers, Wildlife, Old-growth	Swimming, Historic Interest
46	4–5	19.1	Loop	Backpacking, Horses	Stream, Mountain	Autumn Colors, Wildflowers, Wildlife, Spruce-fir	Great Views, Historic Interest, Secluded
47	3	7.5	Loop	Dayhiking	Stream, Mountain	Autumn Colors, Wildflowers, Old-growth	Historic Interest
48	2	4.0	Out & Back	Dayhiking, Horses	Stream	Autumn Colors, Wildflowers	Great Views, Secluded
49	3	5.4	Out & Back	Dayhiking, Horses	Summit, Mountain	Autumn Colors, Spruce-fir	Great Views, Photo Opportunity, Steep
50	2	4.0	Out & Back	Dayhiking, Horses	Stream, Waterfall	Autumn Colors, Wildflowers	Swimming, Photo Opportunity

USES & ACCESS	TYPE	TERRAIN	FLORA & FAUNA	FEATURES
Dayhiking	Loop	Mountain	Autumn Colors	Great Views
Backpacking	Out & Back	Summit	Wildflowers	Photo Opportunity
Horses	Point-to-Point	Ridgeline	Wildlife	Backcountry Camping
Child Friendly	DIFFICULTY -12345+ less more	Stream	Spruce-fir	Swimming
		Waterfall	Old-growth	Secluded
		Lake		Steep
				Historic Interest
				Geologic Interest

Maps

For the Smokemont, Cataloochee, and Big Creek area, here are the USGS 7.5-minute (1:24,000-scale) topographic quadrangles that you will need, listed in the order that you will need them as you hike along your route.

Trail 40: Smokemont
Trail 41: Smokemont, Mount Guyot
Trail 42: Bunches Bald, Luftee Knob
Trail 43: Bunches Bald
Trail 44: Bunches Bald, Dellwood
Trail 45: Dellwood, Bunches Bald

Trail 46: Cove Creek Gap, Luftee Knob
Trail 47: Cove Creek Gap, Dellwood
Trail 48: Cove Creek Gap
Trail 49: Cove Creek Gap, Luftee Knob
Trail 50: Waterville, Cove Creek Gap, Luftee Knob

Smokemont, Cataloochee, and Big Creek Area

Smokemont Loop 303
This classic dayhike starts at Smokemont Campground. Enjoy riparian woodland, wildflowers, and pioneer homesites along Bradley Fork. Climb into dry ridgetop terrain on Richland Mountain, with partial views and vivid fall colors.

Cabin Flats Loop 309
This water-based backpack has a little high country mixed in. Travel up Bradley Fork to dead end at a streamside flat deep in the mountains. Leave the valley and climb to quiet Hughes Ridge where northern hardwoods and evergreens await. Descend to a streamside camp along upper Chasteen Creek. Your return route leads past Chasteen Creek Cascades.

Hyatt Ridge Loop 315
This secluded dayhike leads to a high ridge. Start at an out-of-the way trailhead, climbing along Hyatt Creek. Reach a narrow ridge with views and travel amid spruce. Descend to Straight Fork. Enjoy a quiet road walk on a gravel road beside a scenic stream draining high country.

Flat Creek Falls and Vista 321
This great family dayhike first passes an overlook, and then travels along a high-elevation stream to reach a waterfall and second vista. One of the highest water hikes in the park, the hike is near a picnic area and campground.

TRAIL 44

Dayhiking
9.6 miles, Out & Back
Difficulty: 1 2 **3** 4 5

Hemphill Bald Hike 327

This high country ramble travels the backbone of Cataloochee Divide, on the park boundary. Cross knob and gap, reaching the hike's highest point, Hemphill Bald. Take in sweeping vistas of meadows and mountains.

TRAIL 45

Dayhiking, Horses,
Backpacking
9.1 miles, Loop
Difficulty: 1 2 **3** 4 5

Big Fork Ridge Loop 333

Visit a homesite and huge trees on this loop. Follow Rough Fork in old-growth northern red oak, climbing up and over Big Fork Ridge to Caldwell Fork, a gorgeous stream. Pass the "Big Poplars," massive tulip trees. Complete the circuit with a second climb of Big Fork Ridge.

TRAIL 46

Backpacking, Horses
19.1 miles, Loop
Difficulty: 1 2 3 **4 5**

Pretty Hollow Gap Loop 339

Explore highlands above scenic Cataloochee Valley on this two-night backpack circuit. An easy first day leads to Pretty Hollow campsite. Next day, ascend a deeply cut gorge, reaching spruce forest at Pretty Hollow Gap. Join Mount Sterling Ridge and cruise the high country to camp at Laurel Gap Shelter, over a mile high. From there, follow Balsam Mountain then dip into the lowlands via the lush Palmer Creek Trail.

TRAIL 47

Dayhiking
7.5 miles, Loop
Difficulty: 1 2 **3** 4 5

Boogerman Loop 345

This hike appropriately starts with a footlog crossing. You'll be quite familiar with these narrow bridges before this loop is over. Along the way enjoy huge trees, homesites, and mountain streams. There is quite a bit of up and down, but the trail makers were simply visiting the biggest trees in the area.

Little Cataloochee Church 351

The secluded hike to Little Cataloochee Church is a trip back in time. Pass a preserved pioneer cabin on your rolling trek into the Little Cataloochee valley. View more homesites and farmsteads to finally end up at pastoral Little Cataloochee Church, built in 1890 and maintained to this day.

Mount Sterling via
Mount Sterling Gap 357

This steep trail starts high and get higher, as it enters spruce, fir forest, culminating atop 5,842-foot Mount Sterling. A fire tower stands atop the mountain, where those who climb its heights are rewarded with an eye-popping 360-degree view of the Smoky Mountains and beyond.

Midnight Hole and
Mouse Creek Falls 363

This hike travels up the Big Creek watershed, past swimming holes, cascades, and a waterfall amid everywhere-you-look stream beauty. Big Creek valley has been a recreation destination since before the inception of the national park.

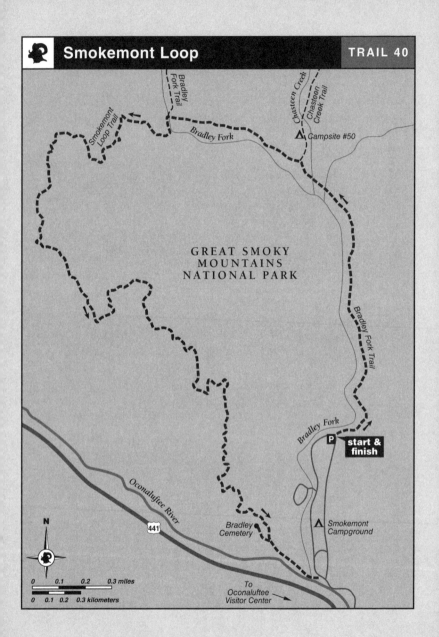

Smokemont Loop

TRAIL 40

Bradley Fork Trail

Chasteen Creek

Chasteen Creek Trail

Smokemont Loop Trail

Bradley Fork

△ Campsite #50

GREAT SMOKY
MOUNTAINS
NATIONAL PARK

Bradley Fork Trail

Bradley Fork

P **start &
finish**

Oconaluftee River

441

N

Bradley
Cemetery ●

△ Smokemont
Campground

0   0.1   0.2   0.3 miles
0   0.1 0.2   0.3 kilometers

To
Oconaluftee
Visitor Center →

Smokemont Loop

This classic dayhike starts at Smokemont Campground. Enjoy riparian woodland, wildflowers, and pioneer homesites along Bradley Fork. Climb into dry ridgetop terrain on Richland Mountain, with partial views and vivid fall colors.

Best Time

Fall hikers can enjoy the variety of tree species along moist Bradley Fork and yet more species on Richland Mountain. The tree variety adds up to a cornucopia of autumn color. Spring reveals wildflowers along Bradley Fork and views from Richland Mountain before the trees leaf out.

Finding the Trail

From the Oconaluftee Visitor Center near Cherokee, drive 3.2 miles north on Newfound Gap Road. Turn right and bridge Oconaluftee River toward Smokemont Campground. Veer left, then turn right again to pass the Smokemont Campground check-in station. Bradley Fork Trail starts at the gated jeep road at the rear of the campground. In winter, parts of the campground may be gated, in which case you may have to park closer to the campground check-in station.

Trail Description

This loop hike leads from Smokemont Campground, open year-round. It travels along Bradley Fork, once home to pioneers eking out a living on streamside

TRAIL USE
Dayhiking

LENGTH
6.0 miles, 3½–4½ hours

VERTICAL FEET
+1,390/-1,390

DIFFICULTY
– 1 **2** 3 4 5 +

TRAIL TYPE
Loop

FEATURES
Stream
Ridgeline
Summit
Autumn Colors
Wildflowers
Secluded
Historic Interest

FACILITIES
Water
Restrooms
Camping

flats. The creek displays superlative mountain stream scenery. The second part of the loop climbs dry pine and oak ridges of Richland Mountain. Partial views extend across the Oconaluftee Valley. The trail winds down to the Oconaluftee River, returning to Smokemont. Extend your trek with a side trip to Bradley Cemetery, where Smoky Mountain pioneers are interred.

Start your loop hike on Bradley Fork Trail, ▶1 at the upper end of the Smokemont Campground. Work around a pole gate on a wide track, making a gentle climb. The ultraclear swirling waters of Bradley Fork incessantly wear away at whitish-gray timeworn stones, stalling where gravity and depth allow pools to form. Riparian woodland of witch hazel, sycamore, black birch, and ironwood, along with rhododendron, rises from mossy banks. Wildflowers carpet the valley in spring. Summer wildflowers are fewer but showier.

Scant trailside forest cover indicates former homesites along the trail. A concessionaire horse trail merges on your right. Cross a wide wooden bridge over Chasteen Creek, then meet Chasteen Creek Trail at 1.2 miles. ▶2 Press forward through the junction, enjoying more Bradley Fork stream panoramas and intonations to reach the Smokemont Loop Trail junction at 1.7 miles. ▶3

The 1931 USGS survey map of the Smokies shows seven homes on both sides of the Bradley Fork between Smokemont and its confluence with Chasten Creek.

Stream

Wildflowers

TRAIL 40 Smokemont Loop Elevation Profile

Turn left on the Smokemont Loop Trail, spanning Bradley Fork on a long footbridge. Stop to look upstream and downstream on Bradley Fork, marveling at water so clear it seems as if you are peering

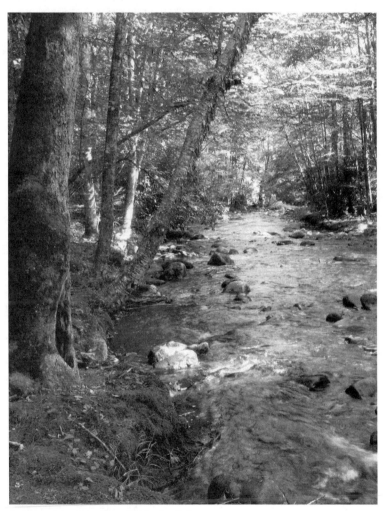

A streamside view *of beautiful Bradley Fork*

through air. Turn downstream to cross a smaller branch on a smaller footbridge.

The narrow hiker-only path makes a hard switchback to the left at 2.0 miles, gaining ground on Richland Mountain. Water sounds fade. Level off in a gap at mile 2.7, ▶4 then resume your climb, now on the west side of Richland Mountain. Fragmented pine, oak, and hickory woods allow westerly views of Thomas Divide. The white noise of the Oconaluftee River drifts uphill.

The trail reaches its high point, 3,640 feet, at 3.5 miles. ▶5 Well-used downed logs invite a rest. The trail then winds down the slope of Richland Mountain, alternately flanked by open woods and thick rhododendron where trickling springs dribble across the path. The downgrade is continuous and regular.

Bradley Cemetery appears on your right, farther along the trail, but don't use the erosive paths shortcutting down to it. Continue a short piece to reach a jeep road and flats along Oconaluftee River at 5.2 miles. ▶6 A right turn here leads up a small hill to graves of settlers, whose names are lost to time, standing beside some gravestones whose names are still legible.

Return to the jeep road and follow it along big Oconaluftee River. Wide streamside boulders offer a chance to relax and absorb the scene. Ahead, an old stone bridge spans Bradley Fork at 5.5 miles. ▶7

The trail dumps you out on the lower end of Smokemont Campground. Check out the campers on your half-mile walk through the campground back to the trailhead. ▶8 This extra distance is counted in the total mileage, though occasional campground section closures during winter may alter exactly where you park.

 Autumn Colors

🔺 Summit

🏠 Historic Interest

🏞 Stream

MILESTONES

▶1	0.0	Bradley Fork Trailhead
▶2	1.2	Chasteen Creek Trail
▶3	1.7	Left on Smokemont Loop Trail
▶4	2.7	Unnamed gap
▶5	3.5	High point of hike
▶6	5.2	Spur trail to cemetery
▶7	5.5	Smokemont Campground
▶8	6.0	Bradley Fork Trailhead

Cabin Flats Loop

TRAIL 41

Bradley Fork

Hughes Ridge Trail

Dry Sluice Gap Trail

Cabin Flats Trail

Campsite #49

Tennessee Branch

Bradley Fork Trail

GREAT SMOKY
MOUNTAINS
NATIONAL PARK

Enloe Creek Trail

Campsite #48

Chasteen Creek

Chasteen Creek Trail

Bradley Fork

Chasteen Creek
Cascades

pool

Bradley Fork Trail

Becks Bald

Oconaluftee River

Campsite #50

441

Smokemont Loop Trail

Bradley Fork

Bradley Fork Trail

Becks Branch

P

start & finish

N

Smokemont Campground

Bradley Cemetery

| 0 | 0.5 | 1 | 1.5 miles |
| 0 | 0.5 | 1 | 1.5 kilometers |

Cabin Flats Loop

This water-based backpack has a little high country mixed in. Travel up Bradley Fork to dead end at a streamside flat deep in the mountains. Leave the valley and climb to quiet Hughes Ridge where northern hardwoods and evergreens await. Descend to a streamside camp along upper Chasteen Creek. Your return route leads past Chasteen Creek Cascades.

Best Time

Summer is good for swimming and fishing. In June, backpackers can achieve a big bloom "triple crown," as flame azalea, mountain laurel, and rhododendron color the trails. The spring wildflowers along Bradley Fork are stunning. The elevation variation is sure to bring autumn splash anytime during the fall. Crowds aren't much of an issue here, though Cabin Flats Campsite, #49, sees summer weekend use.

Finding the Trail

From the Oconaluftee Visitor Center, drive 3.2 miles north on Newfound Gap Road. Turn right and bridge Oconaluftee River toward Smokemont Campground. Veer left, then turn right again to pass the Smokemont Campground check-in station. Bradley Fork Trail starts at the gated jeep road in the rear of the campground. In winter, if parts of the campground are gated, you may have to park closer to the campground check-in station.

TRAIL USE
Backpacking, Horses

LENGTH
17.4 miles, 10–12 hours

VERTICAL FEET
-2,850/+2,850

DIFFICULTY
– 1 2 3 **4** 5 +

TRAIL TYPE
Loop

FEATURES
Ridgeline
Stream
Waterfall
Autumn Colors
Wildflowers
Historic Interest
Swimming

FACILITIES
Campground
Water
Restrooms

Trail Description

This loop travels the watercourses and ridges of the Bradley Fork watershed. Leave Smokemont Campground and make your way up Bradley Fork. Continue to the upper reaches of the stream and overnight at Cabin Flats, formerly one of the Smokies most notorious campsites because of frequent bear encounters. Worry not, as bearproof food storage cables have been installed here, as at all other Smokies campsites. Beautiful Bradley Fork is great for wading, fishing, or simply peering into the crystalline waters.

Next day, climb along Taywa Creek, in places falling steeply, creating a cavalcade of cascades. Switchback up dry mountainside woodlands to reach Hughes Ridge. Here, rhododendron and altitude-loving spruce trees line the trail. Make a pleasant cruise in the high country before dropping to Chasteen Creek and a second campsite. Your final day takes you past Chasteen Creek Cascades before returning to Bradley Fork.

Leave Smokemont Campground. ▶1 Bradley Fork flows, dashes, and splashes along the Bradley Fork Trail, where mossy boulders and ferns lie beneath the forest with many locust and tulip trees taking over former inhabited clearings. Cross a wooden bridge over Chasteen Creek. Beyond this

Stream

Historic Interest

TRAIL 41 Cabin Flats Loop Elevation Profile

crossing, at 1.2 miles, ►**2** is the Chasteen Creek Trail junction, your return route.

Keep straight on the Bradley Fork Trail, rambling through a temperate jungle thick with doghobble and rhododendron. Tiny tributaries trickle toward translucent Bradley Fork, which crashes alongside the trail between sporadic gray rock bars. At 1.7 miles, the Smokemont Loop Trail leaves left. ►**3** Keep straight to reach a spur trail leading left to a deep pool at 2.3 miles. Here, a series of rapids slows to a crystalline reservoir that begs a swim. Look for trout facing upstream in its depths.

 Swimming

At 2.6 miles, come to a repose bench and horse-hitching post. Look across the stream to see a low-flow tributary plummeting 40 feet into Bradley Fork. At 3.2 miles, bridge Bradley Fork as it splits around an island. The gentle ascent continues. At 3.7 miles, the trail bridges Bradley Fork again. The bridge makes for an ideal vantage to view Taywa Creek dashing among mossy rocks to meet Bradley Fork.

Waterfall

Pick up the Cabin Flats Trail in a traffic circle at 4.2 miles. ►**4** Immediately cross Bradley Fork on an impressive iron trestle bridge. Span Tennessee Branch on a footbridge, just beyond which lies the Dry Sluice Gap Trail junction at mile 4.4. The Cabin Flats Trail winds along the west side of the Bradley Fork valley before descending into Cabin Flats proper, at mile 5.0, after a sharp right turn. ►**5** This is the location of Cabin Flats backcountry campsite, #49. This campsite used to be regularly closed for periods because of bear activity, but not so much lately. Whether you be man or beast, I understand coming here to enjoy the beauty of the stream and woods.

The Hughes Ridge Trail used to continue straight here but was abandoned since it bisected Cherokee land.

Start the second day of the overnight loop by backtracking to Bradley Fork Trail, ►**6** this time taking the path as it heads into the Taywa Creek valley. The narrow footbed, overlain on a wide track, first curves around a dry ridge before entering a sharply cut valley with rock protrusions aplenty. Bridge the stream at 6.8 and 7.0 miles of your loop hike. Note the small but incessant tumbling cascades shaded by buckeye and yellow birch. Bridge Taywa Creek at 7.8 miles. ►7 This is your last easy water, so fill up. Several switchbacks ease the ascent, and you drift into a pretty gap with a shady spruce grove and the Hughes Ridge Trail junction at 9.3 miles. ►8

Turn right on Hughes Ridge Trail, walking the crest amid northern hardwoods and spruce. Bisect obvious gaps at 10.1 and 10.4 miles before making a long climb, then drop to meet Enloe Creek Trail at 11.8 miles. ►9 Keep straight on Hughes Ridge Trail to reach Chasteen Creek Trail at 12.2 miles. ►10 This loop descends Chasteen Creek Trail via switchbacks to enter wide coves full of ruler-straight tulip trees. Come to your second night's destination and Upper Chasteen backcountry campsite, #48, at 13.8 miles. ►11 Small streams seemingly encircle the tiered camp, shaded by preserved hemlock and tulip trees.

Your final day continues down Chasteen Creek Trail. You stay way above Chasteen Creek. Watch for a low-flow sliding rock cascade at 14.8 miles. The descent steepens, and you can see Chasteen Creek Cascades. Be patient and continue down-trail to meet a spur trail and horse-hitching post at 15.4 miles. ►12 Here, Chasteen Creek tumbles 20 feet over a rock face. Depending on the flow, the waterfall sometimes splits into separate ribbons as it pours over the rock. The trail widens below the falls because of horse use.

Bridge Chasteen Creek just before passing Lower Chasteen backcountry campsite, #50, at 16.1 miles. ►13 Continue down-trail to meet Bradley Fork and complete the loop portion of the hike at 16.2 miles. ►14 If you prefer a longer exit route instead, take the Smokemont Loop Trail and add 2.9 miles to your final day. Retrace your

Stream

Ridgeline

Backcountry Camping

Waterfall

steps along Bradley Fork, appreciating more of this superlative watercourse on an easy, moderate downgrade. Reach Smokemont Campground ►15 and the end of the hike at 17.4 miles.

🚶	MILESTONES	
►1	0.0	Smokemont Campground Trailhead
►2	1.2	Straight on Bradley Fork Trail
►3	1.7	Smokemont Loop leaves left
►4	4.2	Join the Cabin Flats Trail
►5	5.0	Cabin Flats Campsite, #49
►6	5.8	Resume Bradley Fork Trail
►7	7.8	Final bridging of Taywa Creek
►8	9.3	Right on Hughes Ridge Trail
►9	11.8	Pass Enloe Creek Trail
►10	12.2	Right on Chasteen Creek Trail
►11	13.8	Chasteen Creek Campsite, #48
►12	15.4	Spur to Chasteen Creek Cascades
►13	16.1	Lower Chasteen Campsite, #50
►14	16.2	Left on Bradley Fork Trail
►15	17.4	Smokemont Campground Trailhead

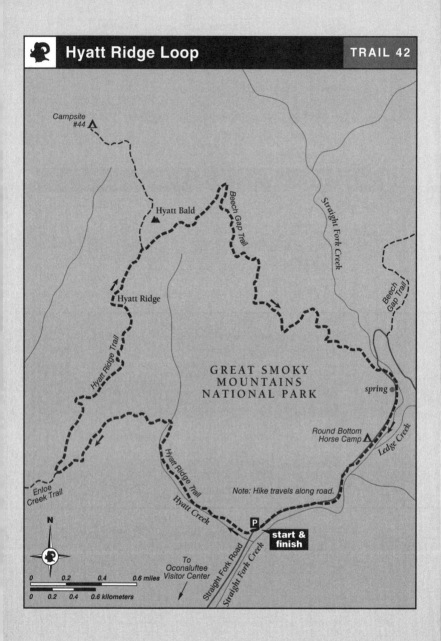

Hyatt Ridge Loop

TRAIL 42

Campsite #44

Hyatt Bald

Beech Gap Trail

Straight Fork Creek

Hyatt Ridge

Beech Gap Trail

Hyatt Ridge Trail

GREAT SMOKY
MOUNTAINS
NATIONAL PARK

spring

Round Bottom
Horse Camp

Ledge Creek

Hyatt Ridge Trail

Note: Hike travels along road.

Enloe Creek Trail

Hyatt Creek

P

start & finish

N

0   0.2   0.4   0.6 miles
0   0.2   0.4   0.6 kilometers

Straight Fork Road

Straight Fork Creek

To Oconaluftee Visitor Center

Hyatt Ridge Loop

This secluded dayhike leads to a high ridge. Start at an out-of-the way trailhead, climbing along Hyatt Creek. Reach a narrow ridge with views and travel amid spruce. Descend to Straight Fork. Enjoy a quiet road walk on a gravel road beside a scenic stream draining high country.

Best Time

Be apprised the access, Straight Fork Road, is gated at the park boundary but generally open from mid-March through mid-November. Escape the heat during summer by going for a swim in Straight Fork after your trek. Fall colors are vibrant. The lesser used path is a good alternative during times when other trails in the park may be busy.

Finding the Trail

From Oconaluftee Visitor Center, drive 1.2 miles south on Newfound Gap Road toward Cherokee. Turn left on Saunooke Bridge Road and follow it a short distance over the Oconaluftee River to Big Cove Road. Turn left on Big Cove Road and follow it 8.8 miles, then turn right on Straight Fork Road. Continue past the Cherokee tribal fish hatchery to reach the park boundary at 1 mile. Drive 2.5 miles beyond the boundary to the Hyatt Ridge Trailhead, which will be on your left just past a one-lane bridge over Hyatt Creek.

TRAIL USE
Dayhiking, Horses

LENGTH
7.6 miles, 4–5 hours

VERTICAL FEET
+1,980/-1,980

DIFFICULTY
– 1 2 **3** 4 5 +

TRAIL TYPE
Loop

FEATURES
Ridgeline
Stream
Autumn Colors
Wildflowers
Secluded
Steep

FACILITIES
None

Trail Description

This loop hike takes you from quiet Straight Fork Road up fast-moving Hyatt Creek into lesser-visited high country on Hyatt Ridge. Up there, experience spruce and northern hardwoods rising over a once grassy bald. A short walk along the lightly used Straight Fork Road completes your loop.

Start your trip ▶1 on the Hyatt Ridge Trail, passing around a pole gate. As you warm up, look for the remnants of an old homestead, including piled rocks, in a flat on trail right. Overhead, white oak, sourwood, black birch, and maple shade the sometimes-sandy track as it moderately ascends. Note a forgotten roadbed below the path you ply. To your left, Hyatt Creek pours downhill in a white ribbon.

At 0.7 mile, open into a rocky cove that is a riot of wildflowers in spring. Step over Hyatt Creek at 0.8 mile. ▶2 This area is a testament to the power of water. Rocks in the streambed are continually being strewn about and rearranged during big storms. Step over a smaller tributary ahead.

Continue to ascend steeply through second-growth forest up the south side of Hyatt Ridge, working around a moist cove running with springlets that obey gravity to meet Straight Fork. Reach

Autumn Colors

Wildflowers

Steep

TRAIL 42 Hyatt Ridge Loop Elevation Profile

Low Gap (one of innumerable Low Gaps in the Southern Appalachians) and a trail junction atop Hyatt Ridge at 1.8 miles. ▶3 You are now 4,400 feet high. Enloe Creek Trail is straight ahead, aiming for Raven Fork. This loop turns right, staying on the Hyatt Ridge Trail. Climb from the gap onto a slender spine of a ridge, with shrubby maples, chestnut oaks, mountain laurel, and galax. The ridgeline narrows, becoming downright rocky. Partial views open east and west. Circle around a knob at 2.3 miles. Spruce trees become common.

 Ridgeline

At 3.5 miles, reach a trail junction. ▶4 To the left, it is 0.9 mile to McGee Spring backcountry campsite, #44, elevation 5,040. The slightly sloped campsite is located by a perennial spring in a sometimes-soppy mountain glade bordered with regal spruce. Opting to stay with Hyatt Ridge Trail to end at McGee Spring backcountry campsite for a picnic will add 1.8 miles to the total hike. To continue the loop, turn right on the Beech Gap Trail. Sections of this trail also have waving grasses under the northern hardwoods, such as beech, cherry, and sugar maple.

The grassy understory is a relic of Hyatt Bald, an open meadow grazed by cattle in pre-park days that is now reforested.

Descend gradually on the Beech Gap Trail, maintaining a northeasterly course. Pass a dripping spring. Shortly leave the spruce behind. At 4.1 miles, in a grassy gap, make a switchback to the right, leaving the ridgetop. ▶5 Wind your way southward, passing the upper reaches of Grass Branch at mile 5.0. Other springs cross the trail. In places, the path becomes a rock and water medley. The waters of Straight Fork hum in the distance. The trail skirts more small branches, to arrive at Straight Fork Road, at 6.2 miles. ▶6

 Secluded

Turn right on Straight Fork Road, as it follows its namesake stream down toward Big Cove and Cherokee Reservation territory. Pass a piped spring to the right of the trail at 6.3 miles. This lightly used road actually makes for pleasant walking. You

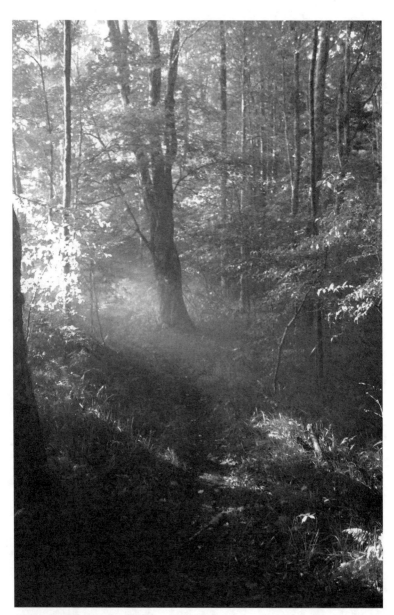

Golden sunlight pierces *the forest on Hyatt Ridge.*

may encounter the occasional person fishing along
the stream. Pass slightly used Round Bottom Horse
Camp at 6.7 miles. ►7 Note the roadside apple trees
here, sure to attract bears in fall.

2 Stream

At 7.0 miles, the road becomes pinched in by a
bluff on the right and Straight Fork on the left. At
7.3 miles, a small stream makes a roadside waterfall.
Arrive at the Hyatt Ridge Trailhead on your right, at
7.6 miles, completing the loop. ►8 Consider dipping yourself or a fishing line in Straight Fork while
you are here.

MILESTONES

►1	0.0	Straight Fork Trailhead
►2	0.8	Cross Hyatt Creek
►3	1.8	Enloe Creek Trail leaves left
►4	3.5	Meet Beech Gap Trail
►5	4.1	Sharp right off ridge
►6	6.2	Straight Fork Road
►7	6.7	Round Bottom Horse Camp
►8	7.6	Straight Fork Trailhead

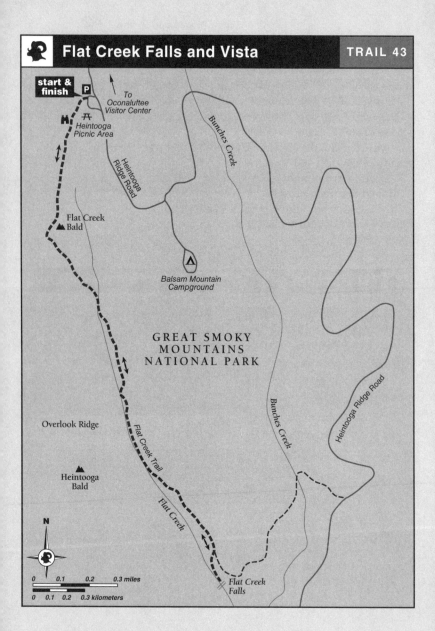

Flat Creek Falls and Vista

TRAIL 43

start & finish

To
Oconaluftee
Visitor Center

Heintooga
Picnic Area

Bunches Creek

Heintooga
Ridge Road

Flat Creek
Bald

Balsam Mountain
Campground

GREAT SMOKY
MOUNTAINS
NATIONAL PARK

Overlook Ridge

Bunches Creek

Heintooga Ridge Road

Flat Creek Trail

Heintooga
Bald

N

Flat Creek

Flat Creek

0   0.1   0.2   0.3 miles

0   0.1   0.2   0.3 kilometers

Flat Creek
Falls

Flat Creek Falls and Vista

This great family dayhike first passes an overlook, and then travels along a high-elevation stream to reach a waterfall and second vista. One of the highest water hikes in the park, the hike is near a picnic area and campground.

Best Time

The access, Heintooga Ridge Road, is generally open from mid-May through October. Enjoy a respite from the broiling lowlands during summer. June offers the most water in Flat Creek and a more robust falls. Fall has colors contrasting with the spruce trees and clear skies for awesome views.

Finding the Trail

From the Oconaluftee Visitor Center near Cherokee, take Newfound Gap Road 0.5 mile south to the Blue Ridge Parkway. Turn left onto the Blue Ridge Parkway, and follow it for 10.9 miles to Heintooga Ridge Road. Turn left on Heintooga Ridge Road and continue 8.7 miles to the Heintooga Picnic Area. The Flat Creek Falls Trail starts at the end of the auto turnaround near the picnic area.

Trail Description

You may wonder why more people aren't hiking this trail—maybe it's because the Flat Creek Trail begins on a lesser traveled road or because it does not connect to other trails. But for Smoky Mountain enthusiasts there are no maybes about hiking this

TRAIL USE
Dayhiking,
    Child Friendly

LENGTH
3.8 miles, 2–3 hours

VERTICAL FEET
+470/+470

DIFFICULTY
– 1 **2** 3 4 5 +

TRAIL TYPE
Out & Back

FEATURES
Ridgeline
Stream
Waterfall
Autumn Colors
Spruce-fir
Great Views
Photo Opportunity

FACILITIES
Picnic tables
Restrooms
Water
Campground

321

path. It starts above 5,300 feet and passes a wonderful view of the Smokies crest before entering high country forest of spruce and yellow birch. The path then descends to the perched watershed of Flat Creek and makes its way to the highest elevation falls accessible by trail in the park.

The Flat Creek Trail swings around Heintooga Picnic Area. ▶1 At 0.1 mile, near a water fountain, come to a cleared view, Heintooga Ridge Overlook. The crest of the Smokies stands north. Field glasses avail a view of the Clingmans Dome tower.

Soon reach a trail junction. The wide track continuing forward heads to the picnic area restrooms. Drop right on a narrow hiker-only path. Overhead are regal straight spruces with their reddish trunks supporting boughs of evergreen, complemented by yellow birch, with its trademark horizontal peeling bark. Cherry, beech, and maple trees add to the woodland mix. Powerful winter winds can twist and distort these deciduous tree trunks. Blackberry bushes grow wherever the sun penetrates the tree cover. Ferns and grasses scatter on the forest floor.

At 0.5 mile, work around the knob where Flat Creek Bald once was. It is forested now, though the understory remains grassy. Reach Flat Creek at 0.8 mile. ▶2 The small, highland stream is easily crossed

Photo Opportunity

Great Views

Spruce–Fir

TRAIL 43 Flat Creek Falls Elevation Profile

Island Forests

FLORA

More than 10,000 years ago, when glaciers covered much of the United States, a forest much more reminiscent of Canada existed here. When the glaciers retreated, this forest survived on the highest points of the Smokies, creating "island" forests. This is the southern limit of this ice age relic. Spruce-fir forests have many more ecologically important components than just red spruce and Fraser fir trees. Boreal plants and animals of the north, such as Canada mayflower, red squirrel and saw-whet owl, reflect the chilly climes of these high country "sky islands." Balsam Mountain Campground is located in a swath of this rare forest. Not only does Balsam Mountain offer the highest camping within the confines of the Great Smoky Mountains National Park at 5,300 feet, it also offers campers a chance to experience this remarkable forest firsthand.

on a footbridge. Keep a fairly level course through pleasant woodland, crossing a tributary on a footlog at 0.9 mile. Rock-hop Flat Creek twice in succession at 1.1 miles.

The surroundings change minute to minute. First you may be in grassy deciduous woods, then under tall spruce, next in a rhododendron thicket. It is all striking. More wet weather drainages bisect the trailbed from the left as the path gets away from the creek. Reach the side trail for Flat Creek Falls at 1.8 miles. ▶3 Turn right here on a faint spur, as the main track continues toward Heintooga Ridge Road. Descend to Flat Creek. *Keep kids under close supervision in this area,* as Flat Creek puts gravity to work on its way to meet Bunches Creek in the valley below. ▶4 Views of the Bunches Creek watershed open near Flat Creek. The cut of Heintooga Ridge Road is visible. Side trails spur on both sides of the creek to the steep, narrow fall. It is challenging to get a complete view of the entire cascade, as the fall is narrow and drops down a heavily vegetated rock

Spruce-fir forests cover only 13,000 acres of the park's 500,000 acres.

 Waterfall

Great Views

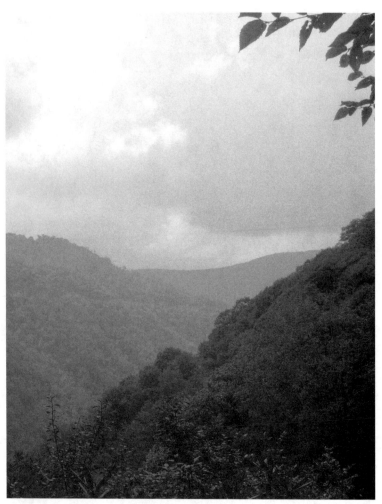

Bunches Creek Valley *as seen from a vista on Flat Creek*

chute. When you are ready, find your way back to the trailhead. ▶5

Consider combining your hike with a picnic or camp out at nearby Balsam Mountain Campground. The rare spruce-fir forests atop ol' Smoky were the main reasons these mountains were chosen as a national park.

Balsam Mountain Campground stands between the headwaters of Flat Creek and Bunches Creek. The campsites are small, discouraging most of today's RV campers. Even with the small sites relatively close together, you will find ample privacy—the campground rarely fills. Since it opens and closes around the same time as Heintooga Ridge Road, it should be open any time you choose to hike the Flat Creek Trail.

🚶	**MILESTONES**	
▶1	0.0	Heintooga Picnic Area Trailhead
▶2	0.8	Flat Creek
▶3	1.8	Spur to Flat Creek Falls
▶4	1.9	Flat Creek Falls
▶5	3.8	Heintooga Picnic Area Trailhead

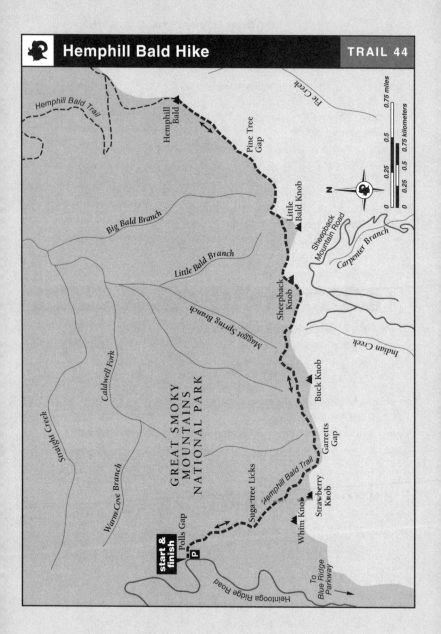

Hemphill Bald Hike

This high country ramble travels the backbone of Cataloochee Divide, on the park boundary. Cross knob and gap, reaching the hike's highest point, Hemphill Bald. Take in sweeping vistas of meadows and mountains.

Best Time

The access for this hike, Heintooga Ridge Road, is open mid-May through October. Spring can be cool and wet, but when the skies clear, you will enjoy magnificent vistas. Summer can be hazy. Fall is the best choice—open roads, clear skies, and good weather.

Finding the Trail

From the Oconaluftee Visitor Center near Cherokee, take Newfound Gap Road for 0.5 mile south to the Blue Ridge Parkway. Turn left onto the Blue Ridge Parkway, and follow it for 10.8 miles to Heintooga Ridge Road. Turn left on Heintooga Ridge Road, and continue 6 miles to Polls Gap, on your right. The Hemphill Bald Trail leaves right.

Trail Description

This hike stays above 5,000 feet the entire trek, as it travels along Cataloochee Divide, which forms the park border at this point, southeast of Cataloochee Valley. Since this trail runs along a ridge that forms the park border, much of the private land along the

TRAIL USE
Dayhiking

LENGTH
9.6 miles, 5–6 hours

VERTICAL FEET
+1,300/-1,300

DIFFICULTY
– 1 2 **3 4** 5 +

TRAIL TYPE
Out & Back

FEATURES
Ridgeline
Autumn Colors
Wildflowers
Spruce-fir
Great Views
Secluded
Photo Opportunity

FACILITIES
Picnicking
Campground nearby

boundary has been kept as open pastureland. This area resembles the Smokies a century ago, when Cataloochee Valley farmers would send their livestock to the hills to graze during the summer. These open mountaintop meadows, or "balds," as they were and are still called, allowed for extensive vistas. The park service has let most of the balds within the Smokies reforest. The contrast is striking, as you discover along this first ridge-running segment of the Hemphill Bald Trail.

The Hemphill Bald Trail leaves Polls Gap ▶1 southeasterly on a single-track path overlain on a wide railroad grade. Beech, birch, and cherry trees accompany the trail as it begins to work around Strawberry Knob south of Polls Gap. Vistas open through the trees, where Cataloochee Divide forms a rampart to the south. To the east, wave upon wave of Carolina mountains meld into the distance. Below you, the depths of Caldwell Fork Valley confirm your perched elevation.

 Photo Opportunity

Reach the gap known as Sugartree Licks, then curve below Whim Knob. Occasional views open in briery areas along the path. Look for misshapen old-growth yellow birch trees in the adjacent woods. Large quartz boulders rise from the ground at 0.9 mile. By now, the old railroad grade has been left behind. The trail reaches Garretts Gap and a fence

🍁 Autumn Colors

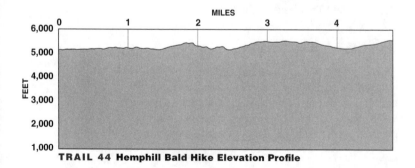

TRAIL 44 Hemphill Bald Hike Elevation Profile

line at 1.4 miles. ▶2 This wooden split rail fence delineates the park border for miles.

From here, the Hemphill Bald Trail turns east and joins Cataloochee Divide, making a steady climb to level off in an alluring flat below Buck Knob. The

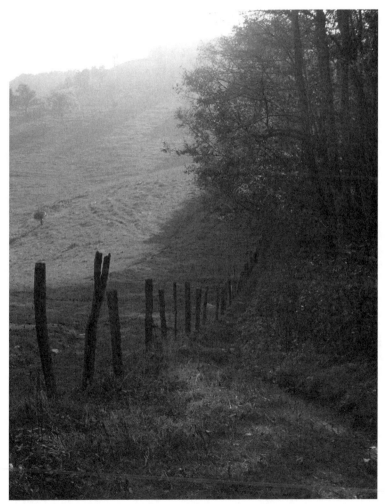

Open meadows *border the trail.* *Photo by Bryan Delay*

path becomes rocky before reaching Maggot Spring Gap, a place with an unappealing name. It then ascends from the gap along the fence line, making several switchbacks to reach the ridgecrest and the top of Sheepback Knob at 3.1 miles. ▶3 The walking is easy in the bushy, oak-topped crest, where upthrusted rocks point skyward.

The trail descends to an unnamed gap. A grassy road ends at the gap on the private land side of the fence. The trail angles up the north side of no longer bald Little Bald Knob to regain the crest of Cataloochee Divide past the knob. Now, the Hemphill Bald Trail makes a prolonged moderate downgrade in a young forest toward Pine Tree Gap. The private side of the ridge, just across the fence from you, becomes open and grassy. The pasture-land presents previews of Hemphill Bald ahead, which is perfectly divided by the park border. The park side of the fence is wooded and the private side is open.

The private land is part of Cataloochee Ranch, originally in Cataloochee before the park came to be. After the park was established, the tourist operation moved just outside the boundaries. Today, their land is a conservation easement and is partly managed by the Southern Appalachian Highlands Conservancy. It will remain as you see it.

Reach Pine Tree Gap at 4.1 miles, ▶4 where there are no pine trees. Begin the 300-foot climb to the top of Hemphill Bald. The trail straddles the park borderline. Views open to the southeast. The area is a study in reforestation and land management. Where there is no grazing or mowing, the mountain has grown up with trees, despite the short growing season at this altitude. And with grazing and mowing, the bald of Hemphill Bald stays open and offers wonderful vistas.

Photo Opportunity

Ridgeline

Great Views

Reach the top of Hemphill at 4.8 miles. ▶5
A stone table, hitching rack, and some benches
are located on the ranch. A kiosk detailing all the
mountains and towns to the east of Hemphill Bald
is embedded into the table. It displays exactly what
you are looking at.

 Great Views

Photo Opportunity

🚶	**MILESTONES**	
▶1	0.0	Polls Gap Trailhead
▶2	1.4	Garretts Gap
▶3	3.1	Sheepback Knob
▶4	4.1	Pine Tree Gap
▶5	4.8	Hemphill Bald

Big Fork Ridge Loop   TRAIL 45

To (276)

Rough Fork

start & finish

P

Wash Ridge

GREAT SMOKY
MOUNTAINS
NATIONAL PARK

● Steve Woody
Place

Rough Fork

⌂ Big Hemlock
Campsite #40

Big Fork Ridge Trail

Rough Fork Trail

Hurricane Creek

Big Fork Ridge

Caldwell Fork Trail

McKee Branch Trail

Civil War
graves

Big
Poplars

Caldwell Fork
Campsite #41

⌂

Caldwell Fork Trail

Rough Fork
Trail

N

Hemphill Bald Trail

| 0 | 0.2 | 0.4 | 0.6 miles |
| 0 | 0.2 | 0.4 | 0.6 kilometers |

Big Fork Ridge Loop

Visit a homesite and huge trees on this loop. Follow Rough Fork in old-growth northern red oak, climbing up and over Big Fork Ridge to Caldwell Fork, a gorgeous stream. Pass the "Big Poplars," massive tulip trees. Complete the circuit with a second climb of Big Fork Ridge.

Best Time

Since this watery loop requires no wet fords, winter is a great time to enjoy it. That is when the large forest trees really stand out. During the warm season, anglers can fish or you can take a dip in the creek. The big trees display their colors in autumn. Two backcountry campsites make a good one-night starter loop, or an extended backpack fishing foray.

Finding the Trail

From Exit #20 on I-40, head south a short distance on US 276. Turn right onto Cove Creek Road, and follow it nearly 6 miles to enter the park. Two miles beyond the park boundary, turn left onto Cataloochee Road. Follow it to dead end at the Rough Fork Trail, which is at the end of the parking area.

Trail Description

Start on the Rough Fork Trail, tracing a clear mountain stream. Stop by the interesting Woody Place, then enter the land of the giants, where stately oak trees form a forest cathedral. Climb away from Rough Fork to meet the Caldwell Fork Trail.

TRAIL USE
Dayhiking, Horses, Backpacking

LENGTH
9.1 miles, 5 hours

VERTICAL FEET
+1,940/-1,940

DIFFICULTY
– 1 2 **3** 4 5 +

TRAIL TYPE
Loop

FEATURES
Ridgeline
Stream
Old-growth
Autumn Colors
Wildflowers
Wildlife
Historic Interest
Swimming

FACILITIES
None

Descend past the "Big Poplars," huge tulip trees, then walk along Caldwell Fork Valley and return over Big Fork Ridge back to Cataloochee. This loop has two climbs, but neither is overly long nor difficult. If you're looking for a 2-mile, family friendly walk, head to the Woody Place and back.

Wildlife

The Rough Fork Trail ►1 leaves the uppermost end of Cataloochee Valley. Watch for elk here. You will have added appreciation for this path when you consider that a road was once going to roughly follow it to reach Polls Gap and Balsam Mountain Road. Back in the 1960s, park personnel worried that Cataloochee Valley would become so popular that it would need an outlet, instead of the current dirt road entry setup. No doubt, the arrival of elk in the valley has increased Cataloochee's popularity, but hopefully its reputation will never warrant the abolition of this trail.

Cruise the wide, nearly level track under maple, white pine, and yellow birch. The valley soon narrows. Cross Rough Fork on a footbridge, then twice more in short order. The trailbed between the second and third crossings is very wet.

Stream

Open to a clearing and make the Steve Woody Place at 1.0 mile. ►2 The wood clapboard structure is worth a tour. A cedar tree stands in the front yard.

TRAIL 45 Big Fork Ridge Loop Elevation Profile

Note the differing ceiling heights, indicating that the structure was built in stages over time. It was once a one-room log cabin. A total of 14 kids lived here, headed by Steve Woody's father, Jonathan Woody, after he married a widower with her own children. There is also a springhouse nearby. The open level area near the house was the garden. Fields once extended far behind the house, and there were many outbuildings. In the 1920s, as tourists came from the outside to visit Cataloochee, the Woody family hosted them. The tourists came to fish and sightsee. Steve Woody stocked Rough Fork with rainbow trout and charged fishermen for their catches.

The Rough Fork Trail enters old-growth woodland of northern red oak. You'll see the skeletons of giant hemlocks, victims of the hemlock wooly adelgid. Cross Hurricane Creek and come to Big Hemlock backcountry campsite, #40, at 1.5 miles. ►3 Camping nooks and crannies are situated between the rhododendron and doghobble. Rough Fork flows nearby.

Big trees are the stars of this loop. Add a pioneer homestead and you end up with a great day in the Smokies.

 Old–growth

 Backcountry Camping

Elk in Cataloochee *are monitored by the park service.*

The hike, which has been nearly level to this point, now climbs away from Big Hemlock onto Little Ridge. The rocky, root-covered trail, open to horses and hikers, makes a steady climb. The sounds of Hurricane Creek disappear. Big tulip trees grow trailside. Top out on Little Ridge near two large chestnut oak trees. The trail bumps up a few more times before intersecting the Caldwell Fork Trail at mile 3.0. ▶4

Turn left here on the Caldwell Fork Trail, and descend through more big trees, mostly northern hardwoods such as cherry and buckeye, into the Caldwell Fork Valley. Pass through a prominent gap, then drift into shallow coves.

At 4.1 miles, reach the spur accessing the "Big Poplars." ▶5 These are actually tulip trees, not poplars, as they were once called. The closest one is huge; it takes many outstretched arms to encircle it. Descend to reach Caldwell Fork backcountry campsite, #41, at mile 4.4. ▶6 It is set in a flat along Caldwell Fork.

Bridge Caldwell Fork on a footlog. Rise to a homestead that was open country not too long ago. Pass the Hemphill Bald Trail at 4.5 miles. ▶7 Keep descending the valley of Caldwell Fork, mostly on a slope well above the stream. Reach a side trail leading right to a gravesite at mile 5.9. ▶8 Up this trail are three former Union soldiers buried in two graves. They were killed just before the end of the Civil War by fellow Union thugs, who actually claimed no side but used the war as an excuse to pillage local residents. Meet the McKee Branch Trail not far beyond here. Keep straight in very level land, growing up with the usual species (locust, tulip, and cherry) that reclaim old farm fields.

Turn left on the Big Fork Ridge Trail at mile 6.0. ▶9 Make a dry crossing via footbridge over Caldwell Fork on the Big Fork Ridge Trail. Ascend on a pre-park path shaded by oaks. Make a big switchback to

▲ Ridgeline

🌳 Old–growth

🌳 Old–growth

⚠ Backcountry Camping

🏠 Historic Interest

the left, heading to Rabbit Ridge. Continue climbing to Big Fork Ridge, reaching a gap at mile 7.5. ▶10 It is all downhill from here into the Rough Fork valley.

Come to a cove and a pioneer homesite, as evidenced by fields being reclaimed by forest. There remains an enclosure used to acclimate elk after they were reintroduced into the Smokies. Cross Rough Fork on a footbridge. You just descended 750 feet. Complete your loop at 9.1 miles. ▶11

🚶	**MILESTONES**	
▶1	0.0	Rough Fork Trailhead
▶2	1.0	Woody Place
▶3	1.5	Big Hemlock Campsite, #40
▶4	3.0	Left on Caldwell Fork Trail
▶5	4.1	Spur trail to Big Poplars
▶6	4.4	Caldwell Fork Campsite, #41
▶7	4.5	Hemphill Bald Trail
▶8	5.9	Spur to Civil War gravesite
▶9	6.0	Left on Big Fork Ridge Trail
▶10	7.5	Gap in Big Fork Ridge
▶11	9.1	Rough Fork Trailhead

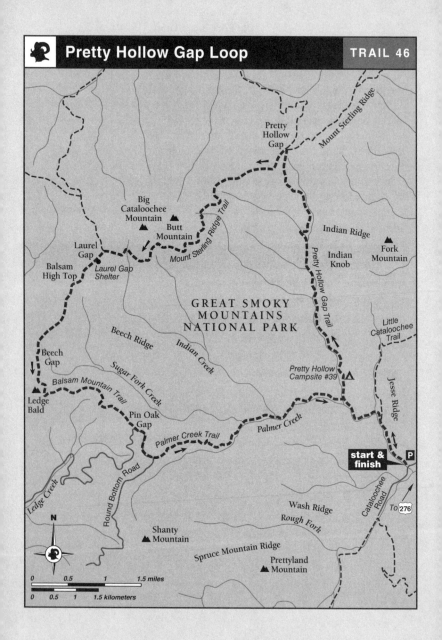

Pretty Hollow Gap Loop

TRAIL 46

Pretty Hollow Gap

Mount Sterling Ridge

Big Cataloochee Mountain

▲ Butt Mountain

Mount Sterling Ridge Trail

Indian Ridge

Fork Mountain ▲

Indian Knob

Laurel Gap

Balsam High Top

Laurel Gap Shelter

GREAT SMOKY MOUNTAINS NATIONAL PARK

Pretty Hollow Gap Trail

Little Cataloochee Trail

Beech Ridge

Indian Creek

Beech Gap

Sugar Fork Creek

Pretty Hollow Campsite #39

▲ Ledge Bald

Balsam Mountain Trail

Pin Oak Gap

Palmer Creek Trail

Palmer Creek

Jesse Ridge

Ledge Creek

Round Bottom Road

start & finish P

Cataloochee Road

To 276

N

Wash Ridge

Rough Fork

Shanty ▲ Mountain

Spruce Mountain Ridge

Prettyland ▲ Mountain

0   0.5   1   1.5 miles

0   0.5   1   1.5 kilometers

Pretty Hollow Gap Loop

Explore highlands above scenic Cataloochee Valley on this two-night backpack circuit. An easy first day leads to Pretty Hollow campsite. Next day, ascend a deeply cut gorge, reaching spruce forest at Pretty Hollow Gap. Join Mount Sterling Ridge and cruise the high country to camp at Laurel Gap Shelter, over a mile high. From there, follow Balsam Mountain then dip into the lowlands via the lush Palmer Creek Trail.

Best Time

Late spring to early summer is the best time to make this loop. The high country is relatively warm but still feels springlike. Fall presents great color. Winter can be harsh and snowy up high.

Finding the Trail

From Exit #20 on Interstate 40, take NC 276 south a short distance to Cove Creek Road. Turn right on Cove Creek Road, and follow it nearly 6 miles to enter the park. Two miles beyond the park boundary, turn left onto Cataloochee Road. Follow it for 4.1 miles until it becomes gravel. The Pretty Hollow Gap Trail starts on the right in a parking area just before the gravel road crosses Palmer Creek.

Trail Description

Cataloochee Valley is enjoying increased popularity these days because of the reintroduction of the majestic elk that now roam the area. You may

TRAIL USE
Backpacking, Horses
LENGTH
19.1 miles, 10–11 hours
over 3 days
VERTICAL FEET
+2,600/-2,600
DIFFICULTY
– 1 2 3 **4 5** +
TRAIL TYPE
Loop

FEATURES
Stream
Ridgeline
Spruce-fir
Autumn Colors
Wildflowers
Wildlife
Historic Interest
Great Views

FACILITIES
Horse Camp

Wildlife

Backcountry Camping

Stream

Wildflowers

see elk pellets along the path. Leave Cataloochee Road ▶1 on the wide roadbed of the easy-walking Pretty Hollow Gap Trail. Palmer Creek rushes by to your left. Pass the Turkey George Horse Camp at 0.2 mile. Pass the Little Cataloochee Trail at 0.7 mile. ▶2

Here, the Pretty Hollow Gap Trail veers left, nearing rock walls and other settlement evidence before intersecting the Palmer Creek Trail, your return route, at 1.6 miles. ▶3 Keep straight, beginning your journey into Pretty Hollow. The ascent is minimal and soon the path reaches Pretty Hollow backcountry campsite, #39. This is your first night's destination. The sloped camping area has four designated sites. A pine overstory shades other smaller trees. The uppermost campsite is in oak woods. A horse-hitching rack is just up the trail from the campsite.

Next day, ascend from the camp, coming alongside Pretty Hollow Creek. Cross it by footlog at 3.1, ▶4 3.4, and 3.8 miles. Span Onion Bed Branch at 4.1 miles. The canopied forest gives way to gorgeous open woodland of beech, buckeye, yellow birch, spruce, and fir with a grassy carpet for a floor.

Make Pretty Hollow Gap, at 5,179 feet, at 5.5 miles. ▶5 Pretty Hollow Gap forms a grassy break in Mount Sterling Ridge. Head left on the level Mount

TRAIL 46 Pretty Hollow Gap Loop Elevation Profile

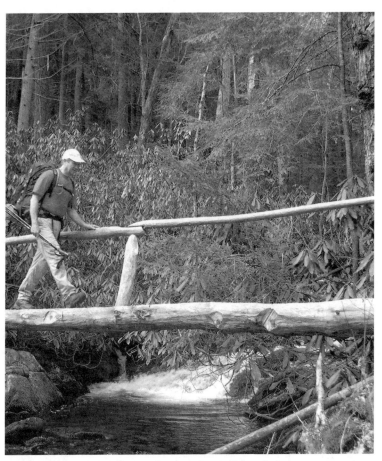

A backpacker crosses *aptly-named Pretty Hollow Creek on a footlog.*

Sterling Ridge Trail. Here, the Benton MacKaye Trail runs in conjunction with the Mount Sterling Ridge Trail. Make a gentle climb amid more grassy woods.

▲ **Ridgeline**

The trail shortly reaches the 5,500-foot level and stays at this elevation for miles, offering perhaps the easiest high country walking in the park. The slope to your right rises high to Big Cataloochee Mountain, at 6,155 feet. Several spring branches flow over the path. The levelness of the trail causes drainage problems in some areas. The track can be muddy in spots as it wanders through thick stands of red spruce and Fraser fir. Bisect occasional open grassy slopes pocked with wind-stunted birch and maple stands, allowing intermittent views to the south and east. Still other trail sections travel beneath rhododendron.

▲ Spruce–Fir

Reach the Balsam Mountain Trail at 9.6 miles. ▶6 Veer left on Balsam Mountain, walking 0.3 mile to reach the Laurel Gap trail shelter ▶7 and your second night's destination. A clearing enhances the highland setting. Reservations are required for this shelter; call before you start your hike, (865) 436-1231. Dark-eyed juncos flitter about the vicinity in summer. This little gray bird returns to the high country during the spring warm-up, then stays in the spruce-fir woods until fall, when it heads to the park's lowlands. This so-called "vertical migration" is its most notable characteristic.

▲ Backcountry Camping

Start day three by continuing on the Balsam Mountain Trail, rising past Balsam High Top before descending through grassy forest to meet the Beech Gap Trail at 11.3 miles of your loop hike. ▶8 Stay with the Balsam Mountain Trail as it heads more down than up, leaving the spruce-fir high country for deciduous woodlands, meeting gravel Round Bottom Road at Pin Oak Gap at 13.6 miles. ▶9

❈ Autumn Colors

Turn left, walking Round Bottom Road to meet the Palmer Creek Trail at 14.3 miles. ▶10 Begin descending the deep forest path on Trail Ridge for a half mile to drop into the steep Palmer Creek watershed, crossing tributary Beech Creek on a footlog at 15.9 miles. ▶11 Palmer Creek's steep slopes prevented the heavy settlement that other parts of Cataloochee Valley saw.

▣ Stream

The name "Palmer" could've derived from any number of Palmers who settled in Cataloochee Valley, starting with George Palmer in the 1840s. He had many descendants also named George, so you can safely say that the creek is named for George Palmer and leave it at that. At one time, there were so many George Palmers in Cataloochee that they had to have nicknames.

 Historic Interest

Stay along the precipitous mountainside above Palmer Creek, crossing Indian Creek at 16.3 miles. ►12 Keep downhill to reach the bottomland along Palmer Creek, where red maple, birch, beech, and scads of rhododendron thrive. Cross Palmer Creek on a footlog before meeting Pretty Hollow Gap Trail at 17.5 miles. ►13 From here, backtrack 1.6 miles to complete the circuit. ►14

 Wildflowers

👤	**MILESTONES**	
►1	0.0	Pretty Hollow Gap Trailhead
►2	0.7	Pass Little Cataloochee Trail
►3	1.6	Pretty Hollow Campsite, #39
►4	3.1	First crossing of Pretty Hollow Creek
►5	5.5	Pretty Hollow Gap, and left on Mount Sterling Ridge Trail
►6	9.6	Left on Balsam Mountain Trail
►7	9.9	Laurel Gap Shelter
►8	11.3	Pass the Beech Gap Trail
►9	13.6	Join Round Bottom Road
►10	14.3	Left on Palmer Creek Trail
►11	15.9	Cross Beech Creek
►12	16.3	Cross Indian Creek
►13	17.5	Right on Pretty Hollow Gap Trail, and backtrack
►14	19.1	Pretty Hollow Gap Trailhead

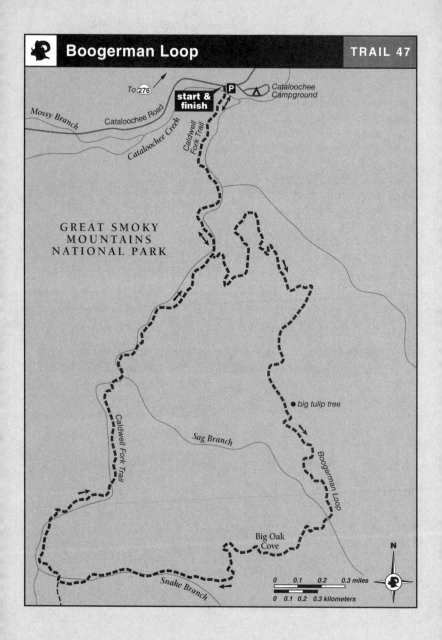

Boogerman Loop

TRAIL 47

To 276

start & finish

P

Cataloochee Campground

Mossy Branch

Cataloochee Road

Cataloochee Creek

Caldwell Fork Trail

GREAT SMOKY
MOUNTAINS
NATIONAL PARK

Caldwell Fork Trail

Sag Branch

● big tulip tree

Boogerman Loop

Big Oak Cove

Snake Branch

N

0   0.1   0.2   0.3 miles

0   0.1 0.2   0.3 kilometers

Boogerman Loop

This hike appropriately starts with a footlog cross-ing. You'll be quite familiar with these narrow bridges before this loop is over. Along the way enjoy huge trees, homesites, and mountain streams. There is quite a bit of up and down, but the trail makers were simply visiting the biggest trees in the area.

Best Time

Winter is a good time, since the elevations aren't high and the lack of leaves allows views of big trees and historic homesites. Spring reveals copious wildflowers along Caldwell Fork. Summer could be warm. The trails are their driest in fall.

Finding the Trail

From Exit #20 on Interstate 40, take NC 276 south a short distance to Cove Creek Road. Turn right on Cove Creek Road, and follow it nearly 6 miles to enter the park. Two miles beyond the park bound-ary, turn left onto Cataloochee Road. Follow it for 2.6 miles to Caldwell Fork Trail, on your left just after passing Cataloochee Campground.

Trail Description

Leave Cataloochee Valley, immediately spanning Palmer Creek on a long footbridge. Enter a homesite just to the right of the trail. White pines are reclaim-ing the former residence. This boggy but scenic flat has been improved with wooden planks for hik-ers. Caldwell Fork flows to your left. Doghobble

TRAIL USE
Dayhiking

LENGTH
7.5 miles, 3½–4½ hours

VERTICAL FEET
+1,020/-1,020

DIFFICULTY
– 1 2 **3** 4 5 +

TRAIL TYPE
Loop

FEATURES
Stream
Ridgeline
Old-growth
Autumn Colors
Wildflowers
Historic Interest

SEASONAL FACILITIES
Campground
Water
Restrooms

lines the trail. Make your first footlog crossing of Caldwell Fork at 0.8 mile. Reach the lower end of the Boogerman Trail. Turn left and join it.

The main part of Cataloochee Valley was a little too crowded for Robert "Boogerman" Palmer, so he decided to make his homestead away from others. The first half of the Boogerman Trail roughly follows the road that Palmer built to reach his back of beyond. There is quite a bit of up and down on Boogerman Trail, and the trail doesn't always go where you think it will or should go, but the trail makers, while often using old roads, make a few twists and turns to visit the biggest trees. Toward the trail's end, along Snake Branch, the path rejoins another pioneer road.

Leave Cataloochee Road on the Caldwell Fork Trail, ▶1 ambling up a green mountain valley. The Boogerman Trail, open to hikers only, leaves Caldwell Fork ▶2 and winds up the slope of Den Ridge after crossing a streamlet. Skeletal hemlocks and gray-trunked tulip trees tower overhead. Continue ascending beneath other giants. Come near Palmer Branch, but turn away, instead climbing by switchback. Curve around the side slope of Den Ridge, full of maple, pine, oak, and mountain laurel. Mount Sterling is visible through the trees.

This trail is named for Robert "Boogerman" Palmer. When asked his name in school, he purportedly hid his face and said, "Boogerman." It stuck for life.

🌲 Old–growth

TRAIL 47 Boogerman Loop Elevation Profile

Turn into the Den Branch valley, where you can hear Den Branch rushing to meet Caldwell Fork. Pine needles carpet the trailbed in gold. More switchbacks lead atop Den Ridge. Cruise along, passing big oaks on a now-easy trail to reach Boogerman's homestead. He thought this place sufficiently desolate for a man named Boogerman. Ol' Palmer did clear a few trees for his farm but as you have seen, he left plenty of big trees for us to enjoy today. Palmer became known for not allowing his property to be logged.

Historic Interest

A wood bridge spans shallow and rocky Palmer Branch. Hike away from the homestead and curve into the next drainage, which was also farmsteaded. An old metal wheel lies beside the trail. Just ahead, at 2.6 miles, stands an enormous tulip tree. ▶3 A short path leads left to this forest giant.

The path passes through another gap into the Sag Branch watershed, curving along the mountainside and dipping to cross Sag Branch at 3.2 miles. ▶4 Sag Branch flows off the slopes of Cataloochee Divide. Enter formerly cultivated timber just past Sag Branch. Note the younger pole trees. The Boogerman Trail climbs very steeply, only to dip into Big Oak Cove at 3.6 miles. Take note of the double-trunked tulip tree left of the trail. There is enough board feet in those connected trunks and the trees around it to fill a lumberyard.

Old–growth

The path leaves the cove and winds along low ridges, looking for Snake Branch. It eventually reaches Snake Branch Valley and reaches an elaborate, squared-off rock wall in the middle of the woods. The trail makes its way downstream in formerly settled country. Snake Branch, flowing off to your left, used to have four homesteads along it. Step over Snake Creek at 4.3 miles, ▶5 and soon cross it a second time. The trail joins an old farm road. Rock walls and lightly wooded, elevated land to your right bear testimony of formerly plowed

Historic Interest

lands. Look right for a trail leading acutely right to a stone wall and homesite, still with rotting logs.

Cross Snake Branch a last time, now on your right. Pass more stone walls, metal relics, and the carved-out basement of a homestead. Make a final descent through white pine woods. Meet Caldwell Fork Trail at 4.8 miles. ▶6

Turn right and head down picturesque Caldwell Fork Valley. Cross Snake Branch on a footlog and soon start the nine crossings of Caldwell Fork on footbridges underneath rich riparian woodlands. The Caldwell Fork Trail can be muddy and confusing; at the stream crossings the trail splits. Hikers go one-way over footbridges. Horses ford the creek. Always take the trail headed for higher, drier ground. Handrails attached to footlogs aid hiker crossings. Since this trail is also open to horses, an accompanying horse ford is adjacent to each footlog, but often the footlog trail and horse ford trail

▶ Stream

Hand laid stone walls serve *as reminders of the park's pioneer heritage.*

diverge near the creek. Other path improvements such as waterbars (logs or rocks embedded to channel water off sloped trail sections) have been added. Note where the footlogs have been elevated with rocks to keep them anchored during floods. Short footlogs cross tributaries.

These footbridges are a dry way to appreciate the crystal clear creek, with its alternating deep pools, falls, and riffles clamoring as you descend the valley. At mile 6.7, ►7 come again to the northern junction of the Boogerman Loop Trail. Continue down the Caldwell Fork Trail, backtracking to finish the loop at 7.5 miles. ►8

🚶	**MILESTONES**	
►1	0.0	Caldwell Fork Trailhead
►2	0.8	Boogerman Trail
►3	2.6	Huge tulip tree
►4	3.2	Sag Branch
►5	4.3	Snake Creek
►6	4.8	Caldwell Fork Trail
►7	6.7	Pass Boogerman Trail
►8	7.5	Caldwell Fork Trailhead

Little Cataloochee Church

TRAIL 48

N

| 0 | 0.1 | 0.2 | 0.3 miles |
| 0 | 0.1 | 0.2 | 0.3 kilometers |

To (276)

P

Old 284

start & finish

GREAT SMOKY
MOUNTAINS
NATIONAL PARK

Long Bunk Trail

Hannah
Cemetery ●

Hannah Cabin ●

Little Cataloochee Trail

Little Cataloochee Creek

● Ola

**Alternate Route
from the South**

Little Cataloochee
Church

Cooks Knob ▲

Little Cataloochee Trail

Coggins Branch

Pretty Hollow
Campsite
#39
⛺

Bald Top ▲

Canadian Top ▲

Mossy Branch

To
Cove Creek Road
and (276)

Palmer Creek

Old 284

Cataloochee Creek

Little Cataloochee
● Church

Coggins Branch

Little Cataloochee Church

The secluded hike to Little Cataloochee Church is a trip back in time. Pass a preserved pioneer cabin on your rolling trek into the Little Cataloochee valley. View more homesites and farmsteads to finally end up at pastoral Little Cataloochee Church, built in 1890 and maintained to this day.

Best Time

This low-elevation hike is best enjoyed from late fall through early spring, when the leaves are off and you can more clearly see the outlines of old homesites and other evidence of pre-park settlers. Spring offers wildflowers aplenty. Summer could be muggy.

Finding the Trail

From Exit #20 on Interstate 40, take NC 276 south a short distance to Cove Creek Road. Turn right on Cove Creek Road, and follow it nearly 6 miles to enter the park. Two miles beyond the park boundary, reach paved Cataloochee Road. However, keep straight, looking for a sign for BIG CREEK, COSBY, joining gravel Old NC 284.

Follow it for 2.1 miles then come to a split. Stay right, still on gravel Old NC 284 and follow it 3.5 miles to the Little Cataloochee Trail on your left. *Do not block the gate at the trailhead.*

TRAIL USE
Dayhiking, Horses

LENGTH
4.0 miles, 2–3 hours

VERTICAL FEET
-700/+700

DIFFICULTY
– 1 **2** 3 4 5 +

TRAIL TYPE
Out & Back

FEATURES
Stream
Autumn Colors
Wildflowers
Secluded
Historic Interest

FACILITIES
None

Trail Description

Secluded

You will likely have this hike to yourself. It has a remote trailhead, and the few people that hike to Little Cataloochee Church do it from Cataloochee Valley. You will be surprised at the ups and downs—never steep—that travel through what was one of the most heavily settled areas in the pre-park Smokies.

From the trailhead, ▶1 the wide roadbed of a trail leaves Old NC 284 and curves down to Correll Branch in moist, rich woods. Cross Correll Branch on a road bridge. Big trees shade the path as it climbs then curves into the Little Cataloochee Creek valley, high on a side slope.

Stream

The Little Cataloochee Trail cruises through pine and oak woods with mountain laurel aplenty to intersect the Long Bunk Trail at 1.0 mile. ▶2 The Long Bunk leaves right and climbs to reach the Mount Sterling Trail near Mount Sterling Gap after 3.3 miles. Reach the spur trail to the Hannah Cabin at 1.2 miles. ▶3 This cabin was built in the 1860s and restored by the park service. A brick chimney adds color to the weathered wood building. Look uphill from the cabin for rock piles from when the tulip tree woods were cornfields. Apple orchards once stretched up and down the hills, too.

Historic Interest

TRAIL 48 Little Cataloochee Church Elevation Profile

Cataloochee Valley

OPTIONS

You can also start this hike from Cataloochee Valley, on the Pretty Hollow Trail, a wide roadbed (see the alternate route on the trail map). Palmer Creek rushes by to your left. Pass the Turkey George horse camp at 0.2 mile. The valley tightens before reaching a trail junction at 0.7 mile. Turn right here, joining the Little Cataloochee Trail. Soon step over Little Davidson Branch, which drains the now-forested Bald Top. The trail keeps up the narrowing Davidson Branch hollow.

The ascent steepens and heads directly for Davidson Gap, which you reach at 2.4 miles. The gap splits Cooks Knob to your left and Bald Top to your right. Descend into the Little Cataloochee Valley, passing remnants of former settlements, which were strung all along Little Cataloochee Creek and its tributaries. Reach restored Dan Cook Place at 3.1 miles. Climb a bit from Coggins Branch to reach Little Cataloochee Baptist Church at 3.9 miles.

The Little Cataloochee Trail keeps forward on a well-maintained roadbed, descending to bridge Little Cataloochee Creek at 1.4 miles. ►4 You are now at the former mountaineer community of Ola. Look for persistent apple trees and dying locusts. Homesite evidence is all over the south side of the creek. Explore the mountain place that once had enough settlers to warrant its own post office. Remember that the remnants are a living archaeological exhibit of life in the Smokies; *leave artifacts where you find them.*

Begin climbing past the settlement toward the ridge dividing Little Cataloochee Creek from Coggins Branch. Reach Little Cataloochee Baptist Church at 2.0 miles. ►5 After you have passed many dilapidated remnants, the well-maintained white church on the hilltop looks even more impressive. An accompanying graveyard lies nearby. Local families keep up the church. Walk inside the church,

Dan Cook Place

If you want to see another intact structure, continue 0.6 mile beyond the church to the Dan Cook Place. Originally built in 1856, the cabin features a stone fireplace, a wraparound porch, and a wooden shingle roof. A short set of stairs leads to a small second floor. The stone remnants of the Cook's apple barn remain intact across Coggins Branch. Little Cataloochee was a big apple-growing place in its latter days. Apples were stored in the stone basement, which you can now still see. Overhead was a storage building.

Preacher's-eye view *of historic Little Cataloochee Church*

and see the wooden white pews and the old potbellied stove used to heat it.

Interestingly, the 400-pound church bell was used to inform the community when someone passed away. The bell would be rung several times followed by a period of silence. The bell ringer would then ring the bell once for each year of the person's life. Locals could surmise by the number of tolls the identity of the deceased person.

		MILESTONES
►1	0.0	Little Cataloochee Trailhead
►2	1.0	Long Bunk Trail leaves right
►3	1.2	Hannah Cabin
►4	1.4	Little Cataloochee Creek
►5	2.0	Little Cataloochee Church

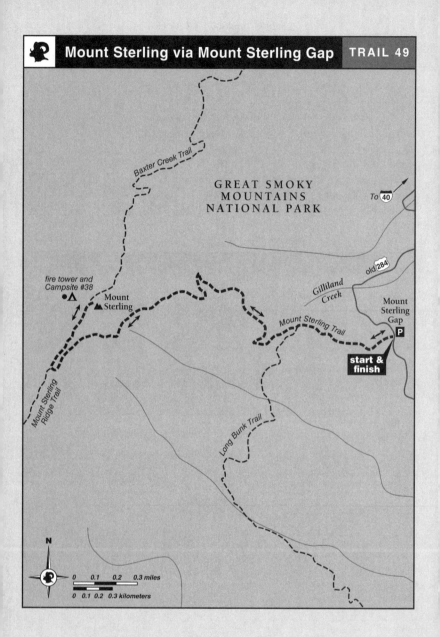

GREAT SMOKY
MOUNTAINS
NATIONAL PARK

To 40

Baxter Creek Trail

old 284

Gilliland
Creek

fire tower and
Campsite #38

Mount
Sterling

Mount
Sterling
Gap

Mount Sterling Trail

P

**start &
finish**

Mount Sterling
Ridge Trail

Long Bunk Trail

N

0   0.1   0.2   0.3 miles

0   0.1 0.2 0.3 kilometers

Mount Sterling via Mount Sterling Gap

This steep trail starts high and get higher, as it enters spruce, fir forest, culminating atop 5,842-foot Mount Sterling. A fire tower stands atop the mountain, where those who climb its heights are rewarded with an eye-popping 360-degree view of the Smoky Mountains and beyond.

TRAIL USE
Dayhiking, Horses,
 Backpacking

LENGTH
5.4 miles, 2½–3 hours

VERTICAL FEET
+1,950/-1,950

DIFFICULTY
– 1 2 **3** 4 5 +

TRAIL TYPE
Out & Back

FEATURES
Summit
Ridgeline
Autumn Colors
Spruce-fir
Great Views
Steep
Photo Opportunity

FACILITIES
None

Best Time

Anytime the skies are clear is a good time to go to Mount Sterling, with its fire tower availing a 360-degree view. Winter can be windy and snowy. Old NC 284 can be closed during inclement weather. Spring has clear periods. Summer can be hazy and stormy. Autumn is a great time, with clear skies and fall colors.

Finding the Trail

From Exit #451 on I-40 just west of the North Carolina state line, immediately turn right on a paved road and cross the Pigeon River. After the bridge, stay turn left to follow the Pigeon upstream. Come to an intersection 2.3 miles after crossing the Pigeon. Turn left here onto old NC 284 and follow it 6.7 winding miles to Mount Sterling Gap. The trail starts on the west side of the gap.

Trail Description

Short and steep, with a fantastic view: That describes the Mount Sterling Trail in a nutshell. Leave Mount Sterling Gap and soon pass the Long Bunk Trail

357

before entering the Smokies spruce-fir forest, found only atop the park's highest points. Reach Mount Sterling Ridge and then make a final push for the mountaintop and tower. Mount Sterling Gap, at an elevation of 3,890 feet, offers a leg up to the high country.

The Mount Sterling Trail leaves west from Mount Sterling Gap. ▶1 Pass around a pole gate, and begin climbing steeply up a wooded mountainside on the jeep road formerly used to maintain the tower atop the mountain. Hardwoods cloak the ridgeline that wends westerly from the Mount Sterling Gap. Larger oaks border the pathway. Begin to run beneath a power line that is going the same place you are but by a more direct route. The trailside trees are kept small here to accommodate it. The result is an open sky and a warm pathway when the sun is out.

In winter, Mount Sterling and its evergreen canopy are visible through the deciduous trees. The path levels and reaches the Long Bunk Trail at 0.5 mile. ▶2 The Mount Sterling Trail resumes climbing and paralleling the power line. The southern exposure of the ridgeline allows mountain laurel to thrive along the trailside here, despite the elevation.

The path makes a sharp switchback to the right at 0.7 mile. Galax lines the trail. The first

TRAIL 49 Mount Sterling via Mount Sterling Gap Elevation Profile

spruce trees begin to appear, especially when the trail curves around to the north side of the ridge. Craggy yellow birches enjoy this cool microclimate, too. Spruce dominates the north-facing landscape above 4,800 feet, standing straight and tall above the splayed rhododendron that drape the steep slopes. Beech trees join the ranks of the northern trees after another switchback. But when the trail exposure curves to the south again, mountain laurel and oaks still hold sway, along with a scraggly pine or two. The forests on the lower slopes of Mount Sterling are heavily influenced by exposure.

Higher up, in the dim of regal evergreens, small Fraser fir trees grow atop mossy rocks, forming a green understory beneath tall spruce overhead. Spring seeps dribble across the path, which passes under the power line at 1.8 miles. The clearing

🌲 **Spruce–Fir**

Mount Sterling tower *on a winter day as seen from Cataloochee*

▲ Ridgeline

underneath the power line opens views of grassy ridges in the distance. The trail then curves right and eases its ascent to reach a clearing and a trail junction at 2.3 miles. ▶3 Here, the Mount Sterling Ridge Trail leaves left for Pretty Hollow Gap in 1.4 miles.

Stay with the Mount Sterling Trail as it turns right and heads north, for the summit. Cruise a grassy ridgeline bordered by thick Fraser fir trees. The path is mostly level before rising to reach a horse-hitching post. Soon open onto the summit of Mount Sterling and backcountry campsite, #38, also named Mount Sterling. ▶4 The grassy mountaintop is surrounded by evergreens.

⛰ Summit

The tower stands at the very crest of the summit. The Baxter Creek Trail, coming 6 steep miles from Big Creek Ranger Station, ends at the tower. The park's eastern swath is the featured view from the

Mount Sterling *offers 360-degree vistas of the Smoky Mountains.*

tower. The main crest of the Smokies lies to your north and west. I-40 and its road-cut in the Pigeon River gorge lie to your east. Beyond the park, the meadow of Max Patch stands clear.

 Great Views

Towers such as these were once used during fire season. Nowadays, planes are used for fire watching. This tower, along with Shuckstack, are the last remaining metal towers in the park once used for fire patrol.

 Historic Interest

Backcountry campsite #38 is a popular site available only by reservation. The favored campsite is in the grassy area below the tower. More sheltered campsites are situated in the surrounding woods. If you are thirsty, there's a spring to your left a half mile down the Baxter Creek Trail.

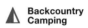 **Backcountry Camping**

𝕏	**MILESTONES**

►1	0.0	Mount Sterling Gap Trailhead
►2	0.5	Pass Long Bunk Trail
►3	2.3	Stay right as Mount Sterling Ridge Trail leaves left
►4	2.7	Mount Sterling tower and backcountry campsite #38

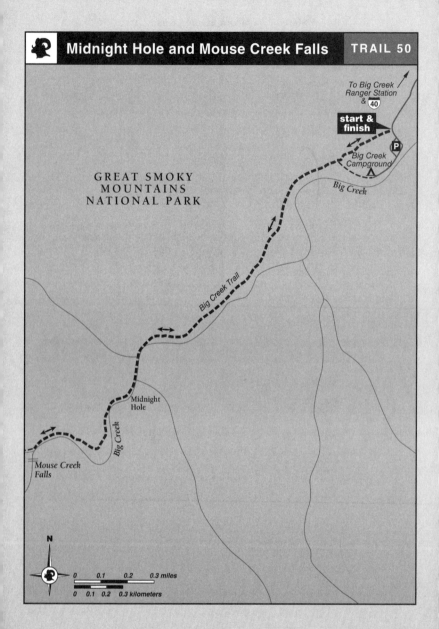

Midnight Hole and Mouse Creek Falls — TRAIL 50

To Big Creek Ranger Station & 40

start & finish

P

Big Creek Campground

Big Creek

GREAT SMOKY MOUNTAINS NATIONAL PARK

Big Creek Trail

Midnight Hole

Big Creek

Mouse Creek Falls

N

0   0.1   0.2   0.3 miles

0   0.1   0.2   0.3 kilometers

Midnight Hole and Mouse Creek Falls

This hike travels up the Big Creek watershed, past swimming holes, cascades, and a waterfall amid everywhere-you-look stream beauty. Big Creek valley has been a recreation destination since before the inception of the national park.

Best Time

Spring through summer is the best period for this trek. In spring Big Creek and Mouse Creek Falls are at their boldest, complementing the amazing wildflower displays. In summer, water enthusiasts can swim in the Midnight Hole and fish Big Creek.

Finding the Trail

From Exit #451 on I-40 just west of the North Carolina state line, exit under the interstate to cross the Pigeon River. After the bridge, turn left to follow the Pigeon upstream. Come to an intersection 2.3 miles after crossing the Pigeon. Proceed forward through the intersection and soon enter the park.

Pass the Big Creek Ranger Station and drive to the end of the gravel road and the hiker parking area. The Big Creek Trail starts on the left just before reaching the hiker parking area.

Trail Description

Big Creek Valley has returned to its original state of forest primeval. Before our time, this area was once home to settlers, then a timber source and camp for loggers, then a place where young men of the

TRAIL USE
Dayhiking, Horses

LENGTH
4.0 miles, 2–2½ hours

VERTICAL FEET
+530/-530

DIFFICULTY
– 1 **2** 3 4 5 +

TRAIL TYPE
Out & Back

FEATURES
Stream
Waterfall
Autumn Colors
Wildflowers
Swimming
Photo Opportunity

FACILITIES
Campground
Picnic tables
Water

Civilian Conservation Corps built trails. Now only the trail, Big Creek Ranger Station, a picnic area, small campground, and trailhead reveal the human touch on this valley. The Big Creek Trail makes a gentle but steady ascent, gaining an average of 240 feet per mile. This grade enables you to look up at the rich forest, out to a spring carpet of wildflowers and into the ultracrystalline creek, possibly the clearest in the Smokies, if there is such a beast. Avid anglers can vie for Smoky Mountain trout.

Proceed up the Big Creek Trail, ▶1 passing around a metal gate, and follow parts of what has been an Indian path, settler's wagon road, a logging railroad, an auto road, and coming full circle, now a horse and footpath again. The pea gravel track stays a good 200 feet above the stream. After a quarter mile, pass a spur trail leading into the valley below and down to the Big Creek Campground.

Saddle alongside Big Creek at 0.9 mile. ▶2 Notice the trailside blasted rock where the gorge pinches the path against the steep mountainside, broken by impressive boulder fields rising up the mountainside. One thing you will surely not miss is the color of Big Creek. Depending on depth and time of year, it displays an array of blues and greens

Wildflowers

Stream

Autumn Colors

TRAIL 50 Midnight Hole and Mouse Creek Falls Elevation Profile

that can almost look tropical. Reach Midnight Hole at 1.5 miles. ▶3 Here, a fall splits two boulders and flows into a swimming pool big enough for an army of sweaty hikers. It's deep, too. This locale draws swimmers during the warm season.

◢• Swimming

Continue upstream. Small rivulets flow under the trail and into Big Creek. Mini-wood bridges allow dry passage for hikers and horsemen. Flanks of rhododendron border the pathway. Take a second to look over now-nearby Big Creek. Midstream boulders have been worn smooth by thousands upon thousands of years of Big Creek following gravity's downward pull.

Reach the short spur trail leading left to Mouse Creek Falls and a horse-hitching post at 2.0 miles. ▶4 This fall is located across Big Creek, and is Mouse Creek's last hurrah before joining the waters

▌ Waterfall

Midnight Hole *in winter*

of Big Creek. Here, Mouse Creek emerges as a narrow flow in a rhododendron thicket, then makes a two-tiered descent. The cataract widens on its first drop, forms a pool, then falls one more time before meeting its mother stream. Mouse Creek drains the highlands of Mount Sterling Ridge above.

Photo Opportunity

Backpackers can hike an additional 3 fairly easy miles to reach Lower Walnut Bottoms backcountry campsite, #37, elevation 3,000 feet. This popular campsite was once the most troublesome locales for "human/bear interactions." Food storage cables are provided to help keep the bears wild and hikers stocked with the provisions they brought. Before they installed the cables, the park service had put up metal poles with hooks atop them for campers to hang their packs, but the bears shinnied up the poles. So the park greased the poles, but that didn't work either!

Backcountry Camping

Campers can also consider Big Creek Campground, located near the trailhead for this hike. It is the Smokies' smallest campground and its sole tent-only campground. This walk-in campground is set deep in the woods adjacent to Big Creek. A small footpath leaves the parking area and loops the 12 campsites in the shade of tall hardwoods. Since it's a walk-in campground, you must tote your camping supplies anywhere from 100 to 300 feet. But after that, you'll be hearing only the intonations of Big Creek instead of car engines and smelling the wildflowers instead of exhaust fumes.

MILESTONES

▶1	0.0	Big Creek Trailhead
▶2	0.9	Come alongside Big Creek
▶3	1.5	Midnight Hole
▶4	2.0	Mouse Creek Falls

Local Resources

National Park Service

Great Smoky Mountains National Park
107 Park Headquarters Road
Gatlinburg, TN 37738
(865) 436-1200
www.nps.gov/grsm
A wealth of information is available on the park's website. They even have multimedia presentations about the park (www.nps.gov/grsm/photosmulti-media/multimedia). If you can't find it on the website, call the main park number and follow the prompts.

Other Smoky Mountains National Park Area Resources

Nantahala National Forest
1070 Massey Branch Road
Robbinsville, NC 28771
(828) 479-6431
www.fs.usda.gov/nfsnc
Smokies visitors often use the Nantahala National Forest, which borders the Smokies on its south side, especially near Fontana Lake.

Fontana Marina
300 Woods Road
P.O. Box 68
Fontana Dam, NC 28733
(828) 498-2211
www.fontanavillage.com/marina
Access the south side of the Smokies using shuttles from this marina. Fontana Village also has varied overnight accommodations.

Gatlinburg Visitors and Convention Bureau
811 East Parkway
P.O. Box 527
Gatlinburg, TN 37738
(800) 588-1817
www.gatlinburg.com
Learn everything you ever wanted to know about the Tennessee Smokies gateway town.

Cherokee, North Carolina, Information
498 Tsali Boulevard
Cherokee, NC 28719
(800) 438-1601
www.cherokee-nc.com
This Cherokee tribal website details the wealth of indoor and outdoor recreation activities on the Cherokee Indian Reservation, located on the south side of the park.

Smokies Partnership Groups

Great Smoky Mountains Association
115 Park Headquarters Road
Gatlinburg, TN 37738
(865) 436-7318
www.thegreatsmokymountains.org
Established in 1953, this group helps the park "through sales, labor, donations, and volunteer efforts, and provides the National Park Service with additional tools for fulfilling its mission." The group, that I belong to, supports the park's educational, scientific, and historical programs, enhancing public enjoyment and understanding of Great Smoky Mountains National Park.

Friends of the Smokies
P.O. Box 1660
Kodak, TN 37764
(865) 932-4794
www.friendsofthesmokies.org
Friends of the Great Smoky Mountains National Park assists the National Park Service in its mission to preserve and protect the Great Smoky Mountains National Park by raising funds and public awareness and providing volunteers for needed projects. They work closely with the park service to bring desired projects to reality.

Useful Sources

Books

The Great Smoky Mountains Association produces a wealth of books on specific subjects pertaining to the Great Smoky Mountains National Park. Browse at: **www.smokiesstore.org.** And part of your purchase goes to support the park. Titles cover just about every park-related subject you can imagine. Here's a sampling: *Smokies Road Guide, Mountain People & Life, Place Names of the Smokies, Wildflowers of the Smokies, Ferns of the Smokies,* and *Churches of the Smokies.*

Maps

Great Smoky Mountains National Park produces a paper trail map for a nominal fee. Buy it at the visitor centers, ranger stations, and select trailheads. You can also download it from the park website: **www.nps.gov/grsm.**

Trails Illustrated, **www.trailsillustrated.com,** produces maps of the Smokies. They have a single map of the park, entitled *Great Smoky Mountains National Park,* and also a pair of more detailed maps: *Cades Cove-Elkmont* and *Clingmans Dome-Cataloochee.*

Index

About the Author

Johnny Molloy is a writer and adventurer based in Johnson City, Tennessee. His outdoor passion started on a backpacking trip in Great Smoky Mountains National Park while attending the University of Tennessee. That first foray unleashed a love of the outdoors that has led the Tennessee native to spend most of his time backpacking, canoe camping, and tent camping for the past three decades.

Friends enjoyed his outdoor adventure stories; one even suggested he write a book. He pursued his friend's idea and soon parlayed his love of the outdoors into an occupation. The results of his efforts are more than 40 books. His writings include hiking, camping, paddling, and comprehensive guidebooks about specific areas throughout the eastern United States and true adventure guidebooks. Molloy writes for varied magazines and websites and is a columnist and feature writer for his local paper, the *Johnson City Press*. He continues writing and traveling extensively throughout the United States, endeavoring in a variety of outdoor pursuits. His non-outdoor interests include American history and University of Tennessee sports. For the latest on Johnny, please visit **www.johnnymolloy.com.**